THE GLYCEMIC LOAD COUNTER

YOUR ESSENTIAL GUIDE TO THE GLYCEMIC LOAD
DIET & PERMANENT WEIGHT LOSS — WITH GI, GL
VALUES FOR 1000+ FOODS

❄

DR. H. MAHER

Copyright © 2022 "The Glycemic Load Counter" by Dr. H. Maher

All rights reserved.

ISBN: 9798356178436

Under no circumstances will any legal responsibility or blame be held against the publisher for any reparation, damages, or monetary loss due to the information herein, either directly or indirectly.

Legal Notice:

All rights reserved. No portion of this book may be reproduced, stored in a retrieval system, or transmitted in any form or by any means—electronic, mechanical, photocopy, recording, scanning, or other—except for brief quotations in critical reviews or articles, without the prior written permission of the publisher.

Medical Disclaimer: Because each individual is different and has particular dietary needs or restrictions, the dieting and nutritional information provided in this book does not constitute professional advice and is not a substitute for expert medical advice. Individuals should always check with a doctor before undertaking "a dieting, weight loss, or exercise regimen and should continue only under a doctor's supervision. While we provide the advice and information in this book in the hopes of helping individuals improve their overall health, multiple factors influence a person's results, and individual results may vary. When a doctor's advice to a particular individual conflicts with advice provided in this book, that individual should always follow the doctor's advice. Patients should not stop taking any of their medications without the consultation of their physician.

❦ Created with Vellum

CONTENTS

Introduction   v

Part I
UNDERSTANDING HORMONES THAT CONTROL YOUR WEIGHT

1. The Insulin hormone   3
2. The Leptin Hormone   6
3. The Ghrelin Hormone   9
4. The Cortisol hormone   11

Part II
KNOWING WHAT'S IN THE FOOD YOU EAT

5. Mastering Carbohydrates   15
6. Good Fats and Bad Fats: How to Improve the Quality of Fat in your Diet   19
7. Understanding proteins   23

Part III
UNDERSTANDING THE GLYCEMIC LOAD DIET FOR PERMANENT WEIGHT LOSS

8. Food, weight loss and Diabetes   27
9. The Glycemic Index Diet   30
10. The Glycemic Load Diet: The Key to Achieving Optimal Health and Weight   34
11. The Health Benefits of the Glycemic Load Diet   40

Part IV
ADHERING TO THE GLYCEMIC LOAD DIET RULES

12. Eating Whole and minimally Processed foods   47
13. Eating Low Glycemic and Anti-Inflammatory Foods   49
14. Avoiding High Glycemic and Inflammatory Foods   54

Part V
MEAL PLANNING GUIDELINES
15. Meal Planning Guidelines	59
16. Vegetables and Vegetables Products	61
17. Fruits and Fruits Products	67
18. Grains	70
19. Dairy and Fortified Soy Alternatives	72
20. Protein Foods	74

Part VI
THE BEST FOODS (LOW GLYCEMIC LOAD FOODS)
21. Baked Products	81
22. Beef, Lamp, Veal, Pork & Poultry	88
23. Beverages	91
24. Condiments, Oils & Sauces	95
25. Dairy and Soy Alternatives	98
26. Legums and Beans	101
27. Fish & Fish Products	105
28. Fruits and Fruits Products	107
29. Grains and Pasta	113
30. Herbs and Spices	115
31. Vegetables	117

Part VII
THE WORST FOODS TO EAT (HIGH GLYCEMIC LOAD FOOD)
32. Baked Products	129
33. Beef, Lamp, Veal, Pork & Poultry	135
34. Beverages	142
35. Dairy and Soy Alternatives	146
36. Legums and Beans	148
37. Fish & Fish Products	150
38. Fruits and Fruits Products	151
39. Grains and Pasta	158
40. Vegetables	163

Health and Nutrition Websites	167

INTRODUCTION

Dietary recommendations have evolved in determining what we should eat to achieve optimal weight and health. The strongest evidence shows that the quality of carbohydrates is essential in preventing weight gain and promoting weight loss. Eating high-quality carbohydrates also helps prevent several chronic diseases, especially diabetes, heart disease, and metabolic syndrome. The glycemic load provides an advanced eating plan that focuses on both the quality and quantity of carbohydrates. People who adhere to the low glycemic load diet may achieve permanent weight loss, improved health, decreased risk of diabetes complications, and type 2 diabetes remission.

The glycemic index (GI) was initially developed in the early 1980s to scientifically determine how foods containing carbohydrates—vegetables, legumes, fruits, bread, processed foods, and dairy products—affect blood sugar levels. Since that initial research led by Dr. Jenkins took place more than 35 years ago, many scientists have identified that the glycemic index represents a powerful tool for maintaining

INTRODUCTION

weight, improving the effectiveness of weight-loss diets, and managing diabetes.

Harvard researchers developed the glycemic load later to provide a more helpful tool for tracking both carbohydrate quality and quantity. Unlike the glycemic index, the glycemic load considers the food's carbohydrate content and gives a more pertinent approach to how given portion-sized foods impact your blood glucose levels.

The glycemic load is computed as the product of a food's glycemic index value and net carbohydrate content. Unlike the glycemic index, it has a direct physiologic significance in that each unit of GL corresponds to the glycemic effect of ingesting 1 g of glucose. For example:

Let's consider a 1-cup serving size of quartered or chopped apple.

- the net carb is equal to 14.3 grams.

- the glycemic index of an apple is equal to 38

- therefore the glycemic load is GL= 38 ÷ 100 x 14.3 = 5.4

The glycemic load of a 1-cup serving size of quartered or chopped apple is equivalent to 5.4 grams of pure glucose.

The use of the glycemic load to rank carbohydrate-containing foods according to their effects on glycemia is the mainstay of the glycemic load diet. You don't have to focus on calorie, protein, fat, or carb counting. Instead, you must concentrate on eating foods that do not cause high blood sugar spikes and keep your daily GL in the healthy range. And, as much as possible, exclude highly processed foods.

Typical low-glycemic diets contain from 50–150 GL units per day. For optimal weight and health outcomes, you should keep your daily glycemic load (GL) under 100. This will help you achieve a healthy weight and maintain your blood sugar level in the normal range. If

INTRODUCTION

you have diabetes, you can eat up to 50 grams of sugar (or 50 GL) from all sources per day (in a 2,000-calorie diet).

WHAT YOU'LL LEARN IN THIS BOOK?

In addition to an extensive glycemic load counter featuring over 1000+ foods lists, you'll also learn why and how to:

1. **choose low glycemic load foods and beverages** more often to improve blood sugar regulation.
2. **plan for regular, balanced meals** to prevent high blood glucose levels.
3. **choose healthy cooking methods**, such as broiling, roasting, stir-frying, or grilling.
4. **choose fresh or frozen unprocessed foods** or canned foods with no added sugar or salt.
5. **increase your olive oil consumption** as it promotes weight loss.
6. **choose foods with no added sugar**. Added sugars include brown sugar, honey, cane juice, fructose, dextrose, sucrose, lactose, corn sweetener, and corn syrup.
7. **exclude Trans-Fats containing Foods.** Trans-fats include margarine, vegetable shortening, french fries, Nondairy creamer, and frozen pizza.
8. **avoid highly processed foods.** Examples of ultra-processed foods include sugary drinks, flavored potato chips, poultry nuggets and sticks, and fish nuggets.

PART I
UNDERSTANDING HORMONES THAT CONTROL YOUR WEIGHT

THE INSULIN HORMONE

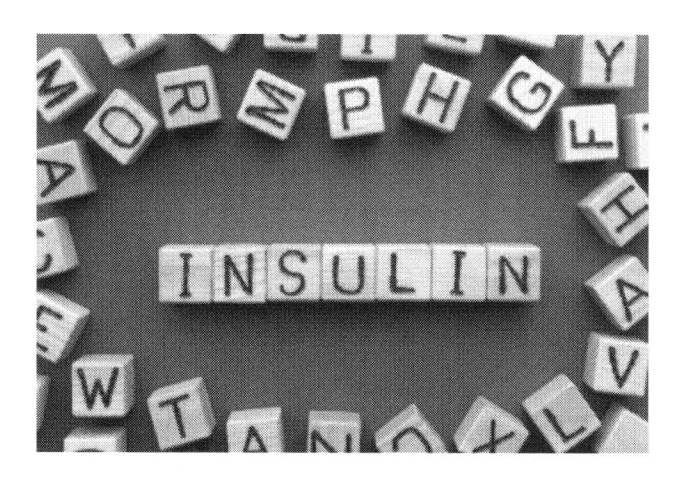

Insulin is an essential hormone involved in many metabolic processes affecting your weight. Too much insulin promotes weight gain, and too little causes type 1 and type 2 diabetes.

When you eat foods containing carbohydrates, they're digested into simple sugars in the intestine and released into the bloodstream. As blood sugar levels increase, the pancreas releases insulin to allow your body cells to absorb and transform sugar (or glucose) into energy throughout the body. As your body cells absorb sugar, blood glucose levels begin to fall to a healthy level.

Insulin also signals to the liver, muscle, and adipocytes (fat cells) to store the excess glucose for future use. Extra sugar is stored in 3 ways:

- in muscle tissues as glycogen.
- in the liver as glycogen.
- in adipose tissue (fat reserves of the body) in the form of triglycerides

WEIGHT GAIN AND INSULIN

In theory, it's impossible to gain weight if you eat no carbohydrates because the pancreas will not release insulin, the only polypeptide hormone that induces fat storage into adipose tissue. And thus, you can not have any more fat stored in your body. **So, if you want to lose weight, it's essential that rises and falls in blood sugar must be as smooth as possible.** The longer the digestion of carbohydrates takes, the better it is. And here came the importance of the glycemic index concept.

Eating high glycemic index food—as you'll see later—cause a rapid rise in insulin level in your blood, translating to excess fat in the body. When extra sugar resides in your blood, the insulin level stays high, and the body begins to store extra calories in the form of fat. High insulin levels imply you'll have more body fat, while low insulin levels mean less body fat. However, recall that too little insulin is problematic and causes serious health problems.

INSULIN RESISTANCE

Insulin resistance is a serious and silent health condition that occurs when cells in your muscles, liver, and body fat start ignoring the signals insulin sends to move glucose out of the bloodstream and put it into your body cells. As insulin resistance develops, the body reacts by producing more and more insulin to lower blood sugar.

Insulin resistance is silent and presents no symptoms in its first development stage. The symptoms appear later when the condition worsens, and the pancreas cannot produce enough insulin to maintain healthy blood sugar levels. When this occurs, the symptoms may be severe, including metabolic syndrome, polycystic ovary syndrome (PCOS), and various types of diabetes.

Fortunately, it is possible to reduce the effects of insulin resistance and boost your insulin sensitivity by following a low-glycemic load diet.

- Excessive hunger
- Lethargy or tiredness
- Difficulty concentrating
- Brain fog
- Waist weight gain
- High blood pressure

THE LEPTIN HORMONE

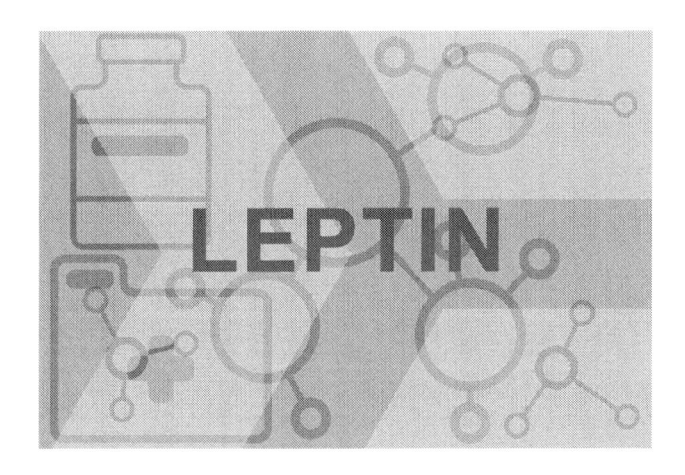

Leptin, referred to as the starvation or "hunger hormone," is produced by fat tissues and secreted into your bloodstream. It plays an essential function in weight regulation by reducing your appetite.

The Leptin hormone was discovered in 1994 and has gained significant interest for its powerful role in weight regulation and obesity. Leptin communicates with specific brain centers to influence how the body manages its fat store. It signals to the brain that the body has enough stored fat, triggering the body to burn calories from stored fat and reduce appetite.

Leptin resistance

Because fat tissues produce leptin, it is released in the bloodstream proportionally to your weight. Leptin levels are high for people who are overweight or obese than for people having average weight.

However, research has shown that leptin's benefit in appetite-reducing is very low for obese people, suggesting that people with obesity aren't sensitive to the beneficial effect of leptin and have developed Leptin resistance.

Ongoing research focuses on leptin resistance in obese people, which stops the brain from acknowledging the leptin's signal. Some studies, however, suggest that obesity induces multiple cellular processes that attenuate or prevent leptin signaling, amplifying the extent of weight gain. Leptin Resistance may arise from poor leptin transport across the blood-brain barrier (BBB), alteration of the leptin receptor, and defect of leptin signaling.

Ways to Reduce Leptin Resistance and Promote Weight Loss

Strong evidence shows that Leptin resistance can be drastically reduced by:

- eating low-glycemic and medium-glycemic foods
- avoiding simple carbohydrates and added sugars and eating healthy carbohydrates (complex carbs, fiber).
- eating healthy protein: Eating healthy proteins can improve leptin sensitivity.
- eating healthy fats and keeping your ratio of omega 6/ omega 3 inferior to 3.
- avoiding ultra-processed food: evidence suggests that these foods compromise the integrity of your gut and the production of gut hormones.

- lowering your triglycerides: High triglyceride levels in your bloodstream can prevent leptin transport to your brain.

THE GHRELIN HORMONE

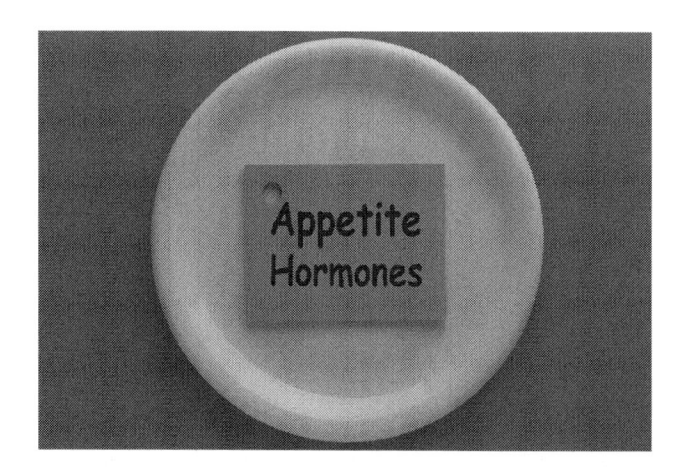

Ghrelin, known as the "hunger hormone," is an acyl-peptide responsible for stimulating hunger by sending a chemical signal to tell you when to eat. Ghrelin is released primarily by the stomach when it is empty to signal your brain that it is time to eat. It is at its highest right before you eat and its lowest about an hour after a meal.

Ghrelin is mainly known as the hormone that triggers hunger by stimulating the appetite. Excess ghrelin increases food intake, promotes overeating, and induces fat storage and weight gain.

HOW TO HELP IMPROVE GHRELIN FUNCTIONING?

Ghrelin levels increase substantially following weight loss which would increase your appetite and promote weight regain. Therefore, you may decrease your ghrelin levels by:

- avoiding added sugar in your diet. Added sugars include brown sugar, honey, cane juice, fructose, dextrose, sucrose, lactose, corn sweetener, and corn syrup.
- eating high-quality carbohydrates (low-glycemic foods).
- avoiding highly processed foods. Examples of ultra-processed foods include sugary drinks, flavored potato chips, poultry nuggets and sticks, and fish nuggets.

THE CORTISOL HORMONE

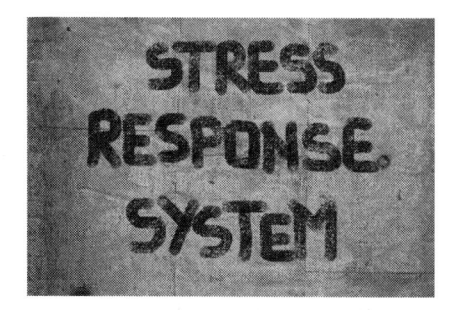

Cortisol is a steroid hormone made and released by the two adrenal glands when the body faces stressful situations. The hypothalamus, via the pituitary gland, sends a chemical signal to the adrenal glands to produce and release adrenaline and cortisol.

Cortisol is naturally released every day in small and regular quantities. However, like adrenaline, cortisol can also be secreted and released in reaction to physical and emotional stress, triggering the body's fight-or-flight response.

Cortisol helps the body make glucose from proteins and quickly increases the body's energy in times of stress. Cortisol is also involved in a variety of essential functions for your health. Most of the body cells have cortisol receptors that influence a variety of critical functions:

- blood sugar regulation

- metabolism regulation

- inflammation reduction

- memory formulation

What causes high cortisol levels?

Stress is habitually accompanied by high energy demand. Consequently, a severe stress situation induces a fast glucose release into the blood, which provides the required energy to deal with the stressful situation. When this happens frequently, excess glucose is converted into fat and stored by the body.

High cortisol levels cause many undesired symptoms, including:

- obesity
- weight gain
- fatty deposits, especially in the face, midsection, and between the shoulders
- purple stretch marks on the arms, breasts, thighs, and abdomen
- thinning skin
- slow-healing injuries

So at its simplest, stress leads to increased blood glucose, high heart rate, and blood pressure, which induces an increased insulin release.

PART II
KNOWING WHAT'S IN THE FOOD YOU EAT

❄

MASTERING CARBOHYDRATES

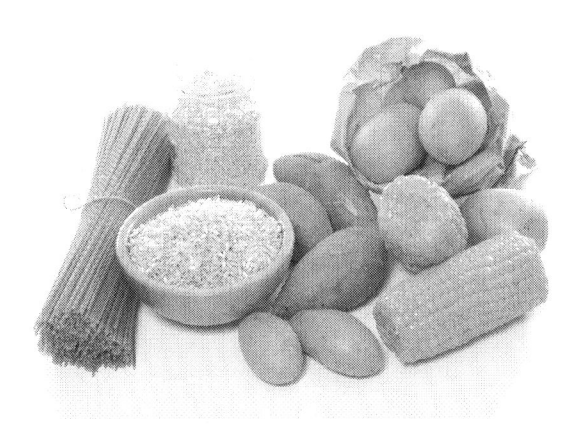

A diet rich in high-quality macronutrients is associated with a decreased risk of many chronic diseases, including diabetes, chronic inflammation, cardiovascular disease, and high blood pressure. Strong evidence suggests that replacing foods of high energy density (high calories per weight of food) with foods of high nutrient density, such as vegetables, beans, and fruits, may help significantly improve glycemic control and promote weight loss.

Carbohydrates—or carbs are one of the three macronutrients in your diet, along with protein and fat. Carbs play an essential role in the human body at every stage of life. They provide energy to all parts of your body (i.e., brain, heart, kidneys, muscles, liver, body's muscles), support the body's functions, promote good gut functioning (fiber), provide energy storage (as glycogen stored in the liver and muscles)

The consumption of high-quality carbohydrates is crucial for the success of long-term overall health, diabetes management, and weight loss.

HOW DO HORMONES AFFECT WEIGHT AND DIABETES MANAGEMENT?

Before going deeper into the choice of healthy carbohydrates, we have to notice that you must achieve the following "Hormones balancing concepts":

- **getting and maintaining the insulin down** will allow you to increase your body's insulin sensitivity and reduce any form of insulin resistance.
- **avoiding spikes in insulin level,** which is harmful to the pancreas and may induce insulin resistance, and increase cortisol levels —the hormone of stress— when the blood sugar decreases abruptly.
- **avoiding ultra-processed and high-processed foods** that compromise the guts' integrity and inhibit or reduce the release of leptin —the satiety hormone.
- **reducing the release of ghrelin** —the hormone of hunger, by eating some nutrients that slow down the ghrelin release in the bloodstream.

KNOWING HOW CARBOHYDRATES CAN WORK FOR YOU OR AGAINST YOU

All carbohydrates, whether low, moderate or high glycemic, follow the same metabolic pathway **that ensures a consistent energy supply to living cells by** breaking them down into simple sugar. They're then released into the bloodstream as glucose and enter the body's cells to provide them with energy with the help of insulin. The problem with blood sugar and subsequently with carbohydrates occurs when the blood sugar levels spike high throughout the day and frequently.

These spikes arise when you eat mostly high-glycemic foods or high glycemic-load foods (a notion that refers to large portion sizes of carb-containing foods).

TYPES OF CARBOHYDRATES IN YOUR DIET

The main function of dietary carbohydrates is to deliver energy to the human body. Carbs can be divided into three major categories:

- sugars: Short-chain carbs found in foods such as fructose, glucose, sucrose, and galactose.
- starches: Long-chain of glucose molecules, which get transformed into glucose during digestion.
- fibers: are divided into soluble and insoluble.

Carbohydrates can also be divided according to their chemical composition into simple and complex carbs:

- complex carbohydrates are formed by sugar molecules linked together in complex and long chains. Complex carbs are found in vegetables, fruits, peas, beans, and whole grains and contain natural fiber. These types of food are healthy.
- simple carbohydrates are transformed quickly by the body

and induce an increased sugar blood level. They are found in high amounts in processed foods and refined sugars.

Consumption of these carbs is associated with health problems like type 2 diabetes, obesity, and metabolism problems. Simple carbs foods are also deprived of essential nutrients and vitamins.

CHOOSING THE BEST CARBOHYDRATES

Achieving your goals in weight loss, weight maintenance, or diabetes management depends on adapting your eating plan to make the insulin, leptin, and ghrelin hormones work for you. The quality of the carbohydrates you ingest is critical in adjusting the level of the hormones. For instance, low-quality carbs (high glycemic foods) are quickly digested and lead to blood sugar spikes, which will play against you and may cause weight gain, obesity, insulin resistance, and increased cortisol levels. Conversely, whole foods' soluble and insoluble fibers (low glycemic foods) are known to offset glucose conversion, prevent higher insulin supplies, and avoid irregular blood sugar variations that induce excess cortisol.

Low glycemic index Foods are known for releasing glucose in the blood slowly and regularly. Conversely, Foods that have a high glycemic index release glucose rapidly. Research suggests that foods with a low glycemic index are ideal for weight loss diets and foster weight loss, in addition to their positive effect on the pancreas (insulin release), eyes, and kidneys.

GOOD FATS AND BAD FATS: HOW TO IMPROVE THE QUALITY OF FAT IN YOUR DIET

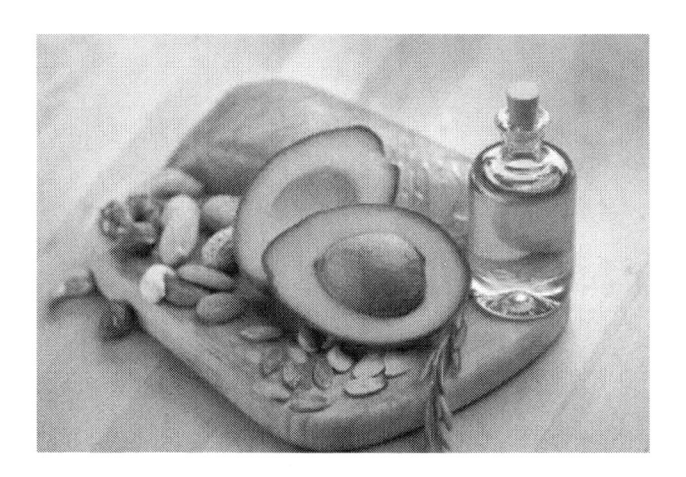

So you must comprehend what dietary fat does to your body, how to choose good fat and how much you should eat.

WHY IS FAT ESSENTIAL FOR YOUR HEALTH?

Dietary fats are found in both animals and vegetables and are essential for your living since they provide your body energy and support cell growth.

Fats also provide some valuable benefits and play essential roles, including:

- help your body absorb nutrients, including vitamins A, D, E, and K.
- help your body produce the necessary hormones.
- regulate inflammation and immunity issues.
- maintain the health of your body's cells (e.g., skin, hair cells)

HOW MANY DIFFERENT FATS ARE THERE?

There are four major fats in food, based on their chemical structures and physical properties:

• Saturated fat (bad fat) is a fat or lipid in which the fatty acid carbon chain holds maximum hydrogen atoms (i.e., saturated with hydrogens). This form of saturated fat is associated with various adverse health effects, while some recent studies moderate the popular belief and question how bad they impact health.

- trans fat (bad fat): (trans-unsaturated fatty acids or trans fatty acids) are a form of unsaturated fat associated with various negative health outcomes
- monounsaturated fats (healthy fat): are a type of unsaturated fat but have only one double bond. Adequate consumption of these fats is associated with positive health outcomes and may replace bad fats. Examples of monounsaturated fats sources include olive oil, avocados, and some nuts
- polyunsaturated fat (healthy fat): The two major classes of polyunsaturated fats are omega-3 and omega-6 fatty acids

WHAT TYPES OF FAT SHOULD YOU EAT?

It is recommended that you eat fats found naturally in food and not processed. Several healthy sources of fat exist, such as:

- Avocado (the fruit or avocado oil)
- Coconut (meat, cream, oil, milk, butter)
- Cacao butter
- Duck fat
- Medium-chained triglyceride (MCT) oil
- Pepperoni/salami/prosciutto
- Bacon fat/lard Beef
- Sardines, anchovies
- Salmon
- Olives and olive oil
- Macadamias and macadamia oil
- Almonds, Brazil nuts, hazelnuts, pecans
- Butter and ghee (to be consumed in moderation)
- Cream (to be consumed in moderation)
- Cheese (to be consumed in moderation)

WHAT ARE OMEGA-3 FATTY ACIDS?

Omega-3 fatty acids are an important family of polyunsaturated fats that the human body can't produce. Thus, you need to get these essential fats from your diet. Omega-3 has significant benefits for your heart, brain, and metabolism.

WHAT ARE OMEGA-6 FATTY ACIDS?

Like omega-3, omega-6 fatty acids are polyunsaturated fats. Omega-6 fatty acids are mainly used for energy, so you need to get them from your diet in the right quantities.

Following different recommendations and guidelines, it is recommended to keep a ratio of 4/1 omega-6 to omega-3 or less, which means that for 400 milligrams of omega-6, you have to consume 100 milligrams of omega-3. However, the Western diet has a high ratio between 10/1 and 50/1.

WHY AND HOW IS THE EXCESS OF OMEGA-6 HARMFUL?

A high amount of omega-6 polyunsaturated fatty acids associated with a very high ratio of omega-6/omega-3 is a constant in most Western diets, including the keto diet. That increases the pathogenesis of several diseases, such as cancer, cardiovascular disease, autoimmune and inflammatory diseases. Conversely, high levels of omega-3 associated with a low ratio of omega-6/omega-3 induce positive health outcomes. For example, a ratio of omega-6/omega-3 of 4/1 was correlated to a 70% reduction in mortality.

Consuming fatty fish twice a week, eating whole foods, and choosing dairy products and meat from grass-fed animals can help you improve your omega-6:omega-3 ratio.

UNDERSTANDING PROTEINS

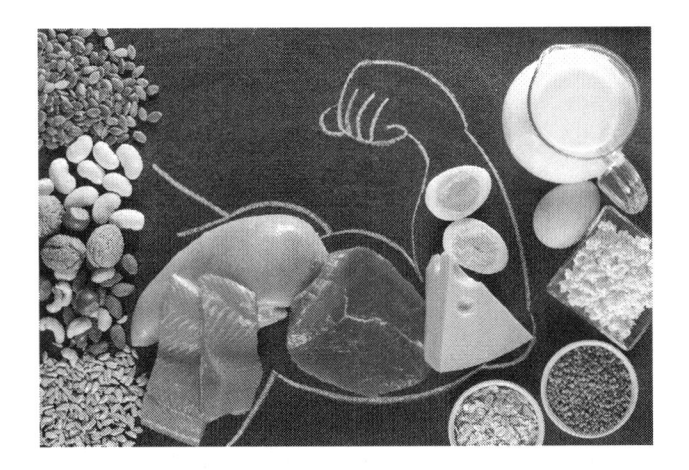

※

Proteins are, with carbohydrates and lipids, one of the three macronutrients in your diet. They consist of amino acids linked by peptide bonds. Proteins are essential for muscle and bone vitality and are involved in building and maintaining every cell in your body. They also intervene in many critical processes, such as creating and repairing tissues, building muscles, blood, hair, and skin, and producing hormones, enzymes, and other body chemicals.

Adequate protein consumption is essential for improving and maintaining optimal health during all stages of life. Unlike fats and carbs, the human body does not store protein, and you must eat an adequate amount to maintain overall health and promote optimal growth and body functions. In addition, eating enough protein reduces levels of ghrelin (the hunger hormone) and stimulates the production of the satiety hormones (PYY and GLP-1)

GUIDELINES FOR INDIVIDUALIZED PROTEIN INTAKE

The Recommended Dietary Allowance (RDA) for protein is the minimum amount you need to satisfy your basic nutritional requirements. It corresponds to the minimum amount to maintain nitrogen balance (i.e., prevent you from getting sick). The RDA must be understood as the minimum you need to eat and is lower than what you should eat each day to maintain optimal health and achieve muscle growth. The RDA for protein is 0.8 g per kg of body weight, regardless of age. However, if you target to lose weight, you should aim for a daily protein intake of 0.8-1.0 grams per kg of body weight.

PART III
UNDERSTANDING THE GLYCEMIC LOAD DIET FOR PERMANENT WEIGHT LOSS

❄

FOOD, WEIGHT LOSS AND DIABETES

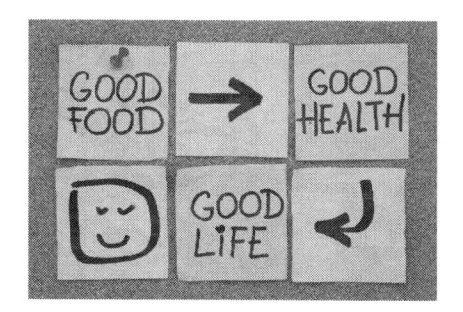

❄

Eating to lower blood sugar spikes is not a one-size-fits-all approach. Different people, even twins, may respond to the same foods differently. However, following the glycemic load dietary pattern will ensure you get the most out of its beneficial effects. People who adhere to this diet more closely have consistently lower blood sugar levels, lower blood pressure, increased LDL cholesterol, reduced HDL cholesterol, and reduced triglycerides than those following other diets. It is considered healthier than modern fad diets (e.g., keto, low-carb, high-fat diets) because it is centered around eating low glycemic, whole, or minimally processed foods and avoiding high glycemic foods.

■ DIET, WEIGHT LOSS, AND DIABETES

Hundreds of diets have been created with many promises regarding weight loss, inflammation reduction, and diabetes reversal. Low-carb/high-fat diets and low-fat diets were thought to be the best approaches to losing weight, controlling diabetes, and achieving a healthy weight. However, a growing body of evidence shows that these diets often don't work:

- low-fat diets tend to replace fat with easily digested carbohydrates.
- low-carb, high-fat diets overlook the importance of carbohydrates and often replace carbohydrates with highly processed fat-containing foods.
- fad diets often overlook the body's fundamental need for a balanced diet

The best diets that work restrict calories to some extent, supply sufficient and high-quality nutrients, avoid unhealthy foods, and balance hormones that help achieve optimal weight, and regulate your blood sugar. Diets do this in three main ways:

1. getting you to eat sufficient healthy foods and avoid bad ones
2. getting you aware of foods and nutrients you should include in your diet to achieve weight loss, better diabetes control, and prevent complications.
3. changing some of your bad eating habits and the ways you consider highly processed foods and refined carbohydrates

The best diet for losing weight and/or diabetes control is one that is good for all body parts, from your brain to your heart to your pancreas. It is also a diet you can embrace and live with for a long time. In other words, a powerful diet rooted in nature that offers a flexible eating pattern provides healthy choices, banishes unhealthy foods, and doesn't require an extensive (and probably expensive) shopping list or supplements.

A healthy balanced diet with sufficient and adequate nutritional elements is critical for battling diabetes, weight gain, and obesity. Both nutritional deficiency and excess are tied with diseases and poor health conditions. Nutritional excess, particularly in highly-processed foods, refined carbohydrates, saturated fats, trans-fatty acids, sugar-sweetened foods, and sodium, can result in severe chronic inflammatory illnesses such as autoimmune disease, cardiovascular disease, bone disorders, diabetes as well as obesity. In contrast, nutritional deficiencies can lead to impairments of body function, fatigue, and conditions associated with vitamin and mineral deficiencies.

One diet that allows that is a Low glycemic load type diet. Such a diet —and its many variations—usually include:

- **several servings of plant foods** (e.g., vegetables, fruits) a day
- **whole and minimally processed foods**
- **a daily serving of seeds and nuts**
- **healthy fats and oils high in omega-3 fatty acids** (olive oil, canola, cod liver oil, fatty fish, flaxseed oil, Walnut oil, sunflower oil, etc.)
- **lean protein mainly from fish, poultry, and nuts**
- **limited amounts of sodium**
- **very limited quantities of refined carbohydrates** (e.g., white flour, white rice, white sugar, brown sugar, honey, corn syrup)
- **limited alcoholic drinks**
- **NO high glycemic load foods**
- **NO trans fats**
- **NO highly processed foods**

THE GLYCEMIC INDEX DIET

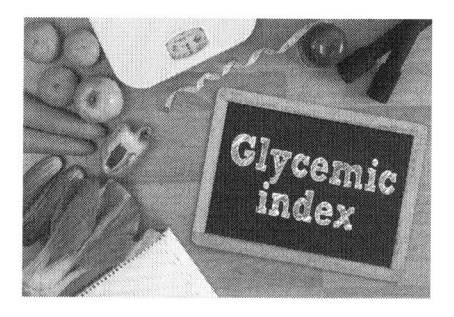

THE GLYCEMIC INDEX DIET

The glycemic index concept was developed in the early 1980s to determine how carbohydrate-containing foods affect blood sugar levels scientifically. Since that initial research led by Dr. Jenkins took place more than 35 years ago, many scientists have identified that the glycemic index (GI) can be a powerful tool for maintaining weight, improving the effectiveness of weight-loss diets, and managing diabetes.

The glycemic index isn't formally a diet in the sense that you have to conform to strict rules, follow particular meal plans or eliminate some foods from your daily meals. Instead, it's a scientific method of identifying how carbohydrates in foods affect blood sugar levels and measuring how slowly or quickly they raise blood sugar. Thus, the Glycemic Index referential is particularly important to know if you want to maintain weight, lose weight, take more control of diabetes, and fix some specific health issues.

The "glycemic index (GI) diet" refers to a targeted diet plan that uses the glycemic index as the primary and only guides for meal planning. Unlike other diet plans that provide a strict recommendation with a specific ratio, the glycemic index diet (GI diet) doesn't specify the optimal daily number of calories, carbohydrates, protein, or fats for weight maintenance or weight loss. Instead, it provides an effective eating plan with more flexibility and sustainable results in weight loss, weight management, and diabetes control.

UNDERSTANDING GI VALUES

Glycemic index (GI) values are divided into three categories:

- low GI: This category comprises foods that have their GI value below 55
- medium GI: This category comprises foods that have their GI value in the range of 56 to 69
- high GI: In general, this category must be avoided because foods cause high spikes in the blood sugar level. Their GI values are equal to or higher to 70

Low GI vs. High GI Foods

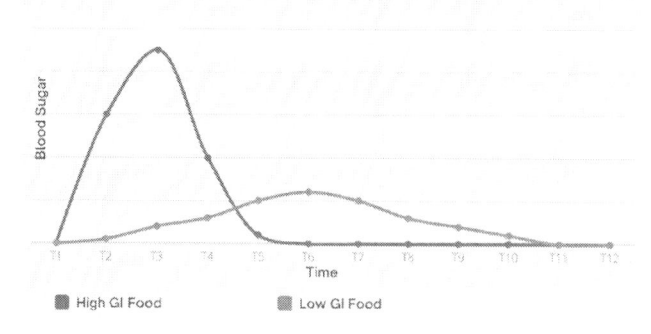

Comparing the GI values may help guide your food choices. For example, muesli has a GI value of approximately 86. A vegetable and fruit smoothie drink has a GI value of 55.

HOW DOES GLYCEMIC INDEX (GI) DIET WORK?

Eating according to the Glycemic Index Diet looks simple because all you need to know is where different foods fall on the 0 to 100 glycemic index (GI).

- You fill up on low GI foods (GI value: 55 and under)
- Eat smaller amounts of medium GI foods (GI value: 56 to 69)
- And mostly avoid high GI foods (GI value: 70 and up)

Besides referring to the glycemic index lists as needed, there is no complex weighing or measuring and no need to track your calorie intake. However, you will have to concoct your eating plan and menus yourself.

HOW IS GLYCEMIC INDEX MEASURED?

Glycemic Index values of foods are measured using valid and proven scientific methods. GI values cannot be easily guessed just by looking at the composition of specific food or the nutrition facts on food packaging.

The GI measurement Follows the international standard method and provides commonly accepted values. (GI values can also be estimated with a good approximation through advanced data science tools.)

The Glycemic Index value of food is measured by feeding over ten healthy people a portion of the food object of the study and containing fifty grams of digestible carbohydrate and then measuring the effect for each participant on his blood glucose levels (blood glucose response) over the next two hours.

The second part of the process consists of giving the same participants an equal carbohydrate portion of the glucose (used as the reference food) and measuring their blood glucose response over the next two hours.

The Glycemic Index value for the food is then calculated for each participant by using a simple formula (dividing the blood glucose response for the food by their blood glucose response for the glucose (reference food)). The final value of the food's Glycemic Index is the average value for the participants (over 10).

Carbohydrates with a low GI value (55 or less) are more slowly digested, absorbed, and metabolized and induce a smaller and slower rise in blood glucose and, therefore, usually, insulin levels.

Low glycemic diets or foods are associated with a reduced risk of chronic disease. Low glycemic index foods are known to release glucose in the blood slowly and regularly. Conversely, Foods that have a high glycemic index are known for their property of releasing glucose rapidly. Researches suggest that foods with a low glycemic index (LGI foods) are ideal for weight loss diets and foster lasting weight loss, in addition to their positive effect on the pancreas (insulin release), eyes, and kidney.

THE GLYCEMIC LOAD DIET: THE KEY TO ACHIEVING OPTIMAL HEALTH AND WEIGHT

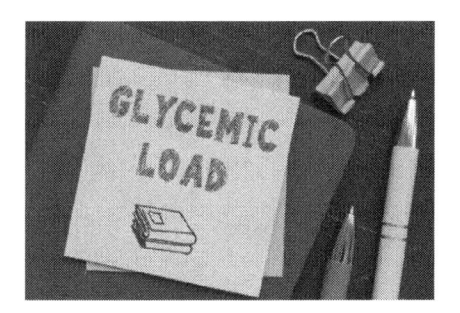

The glycemic index provides a valuable tool to assess how carbohydrate-containing food affects your blood sugar. However, it doesn't inform you how high your blood sugar will go when you eat that food. The glycemic load was developed to provide a complete picture. It tells about how the food affects your blood sugar and how much pure glucose per serving it delivers.

Harvard researchers developed the glycemic load to provide a more helpful tool for tracking both carbohydrates' quality and quantity. The glycemic load of a specific food—computed as the product of that food's glycemic index value and its net carbohydrate content —has direct physiologic significance in that each unit of GL corresponds to the glycemic effect of ingesting 1 g of pure glucose. Typical low-glycemic diets contain from 50–150 GL units per day. For positive health outcomes, it is recommended to keep your daily glycemic load under 100. This will help keep your A1C level in the normal range and achieve a healthy weight if you are overweight or obese.

People with diabetes can eat up to 50 grams of sugar from all sources per day (in a 2,000-calorie diet). This means that you should target a GL of 50.

The Glycemic Load (GL) is computed using the following formula:

Glycemic Load (GL) = GI x Net Carbohydrates (grams) content per portion ÷ 100

Where net carbohydrate = total carbohydrates - dietary fiber

One unit of GL corresponds to the glycemic effect of ingesting 1 g of glucose. Typical low glycemic load diets contain 80–150 GL units per day.

Eating a portion of food with a GL of 10 is equivalent to ingesting 10 grams of glucose.

For example:

Let's consider a 1-cup serving size of quartered or chopped apple.

- net carb or available carbohydrate is equal to 14.3 grams.
- the glycemic index of an apple is equal to 38
- therefore the glycemic load is GL= 38 ÷ 100 x 14.3 = 5.4

The glycemic load of a 1-cup serving size of quartered or chopped apple is equivalent to 5.4 grams of pure glucose.

THE GLYCEMIC LOAD RANGES

Like the glycemic index, the glycemic load (GL) of a food can be classified as:

- **low:** 10 or less
- **medium:** 11 – 19
- **high:** 20 or more

For a standard serving size of food, glycemic load (GL) is considered high with GL greater or equal to 20, medium with GL in the range of 11-19, and low with GL less or equal to 10. The Daily GL is the sum of the GL values for all foods consumed during the day.

As shown in the formula, the GL of a food is a product of 2 factors: the GI of the food and the net carb in food for a given serving size. And therefore, to increase or decrease GL, you must act primarily on the serving size. For example, medium-to-high GI foods like wheat bran bagel, barely bread, and watermelon have low GLs.

Eating many high glycemic foods frequently increases the risk of diabetes complications, cardiovascular disease, and obesity. Conversely, eating low glycemic foods has been shown to help control type 2 diabetes, improve blood markers and improve weight loss.

Because there is a gap in the GL ranges, a food with a glycemic load (GL) of 10.1 is considered a medium GL. A food with a glycemic load (GL) of 19.1 is considered a High GL.

THE GLYCEMIC LOAD OF A MIXED MEAL

Combining foods with different glycemic load values together in one meal means creating a new glycemic load for the mixed meal. You can easily understand that measuring the new GL is a challenging task. However, you can estimate this value easily by using the GL values of individual foods since one GL corresponds to ingesting 1 g of pure glucose.

The glycemic load of a meal can be obtained by adding the GL values of foods.

FACTORS AFFECTING A FOOD'S GLYCEMIC LOAD

Many factors affect the glycemic load of food. These factors include:

Food Processing Methods: Food processing has been practiced for centuries in the form of cooking, dehydrating, fermenting, ultraviolet radiation, and salt preservation. However, modern food processing methods are more sophisticated and complex and alter foods considerably by adding many ingredients, including trans fats, high-fructose corn syrup, salts, artificial sweeteners, flavors, colors, and other chemical additives. The US Department of Agriculture (USDA) defines processed food as one that has undergone any procedure that alters it from its natural state. Highly Processed foods generally have a higher glycemic index and glycemic load because they contain added sugar and are so refined that you digest them more quickly than minimally processed alternatives.

Cooking methods: Cooking time significantly affects the GL measurement. Strong evidence indicates that the more cooked the food, the higher the GI and the GL. Pasta cooked al dente has a lower GL and GI than pasta boiled until soft. Adding fat, lemon juice, or vinegar to a meal recipe also decreases its GI and GL values.

Ripeness: when fruits or vegetables ripen, their nutritional compositions change significantly. Sugar content increases as the fruit or starchy vegetables mature as part of the ripening process. The starch in fruits or vegetables is transformed into sugars, and the proportion of simple sugar rises to roughly 20%. Therefore, ripe and over-ripe foods generally have a higher glycemic index and load than unripe foods.

Physical form: Complex carbohydrates are formed by sugar molecules linked together in complex and long chains. Complex carbohydrates are digested slowly and do not cause high spikes in your blood sugar. Conversely, the body quickly transforms simple or refined carbohydrates and induces powerful blood sugar spikes. Therefore, refined and simple carbohydrate-containing foods generally have a higher glycemic index and load than complex carbs.

SHOULD PEOPLE WITH DIABETES EAT A GLYCEMIC LOAD DIET?

Whereas the glycemic index is a good tool for making good food choices, the glycemic load goes beyond and helps to determine how different portion sizes of different foods compare. It allows you to eat the right serving sizes that would not cause high blood sugar spikes and would not release too much glucose in your bloodstream.

WILL GLYCEMIC LOAD DIET HELP YOU LOSE WEIGHT?

Low-glycemic diets demonstrate much more short-term and midterm weight loss than other diets. Eating low glycemic load foods and keeping your daily glycemic load under 100 is the key to weight loss and hormonal balance. A 2012-study published in the Journal of "The American Medical Association" found low glycemic diets to be best and superior at maintaining weight loss compared to very low carbohydrate diets (like the ketogenic or keto diet) and low-fat diets. The findings support the low glycemic diet's assumption that "a calorie is not a calorie" and that "different kinds of food will affect us in different ways, despite having the same calorie number." Another 2014-study published in "The American Journal of Clinical Nutrition" supports low Glycemic and calorie-restricted diets as more effective than high Glycemic Index and low-fat diets for weight management and weight loss.

■ LIMITATIONS OF THE CONCEPT

The glycemic index and glycemic load are great tools, but they do have a few limitations that you need to know:

- the lists of GI are quite limited. GI testing is new, and the process is expensive, time and resource-consuming.
- the glycemic index depends on some external intervention like cooking. Al Dente Pasta is known to have a Lower Glycemic Index
- the testing results may vary. As explained in the previous section, researchers rely on observing tests involving participants' metabolism to measure the glycemic index. This explains why GI may vary among studies.

Despite these limitations, the glycemic load diet provides handy tools that will help you achieve your goals in terms of diabetes control, diabetes complications prevention, and weight loss.

THE HEALTH BENEFITS OF THE GLYCEMIC LOAD DIET

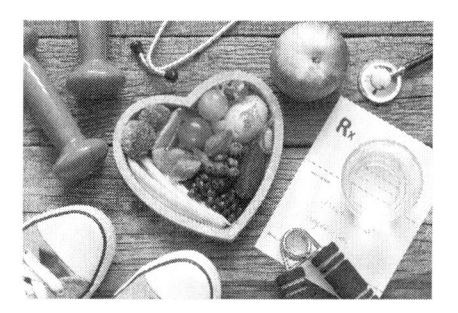

High insulin levels caused by high glycemic index foods are harmful and promote long-term high blood fat, high blood glucose, and high blood pressure and increase the risk of a heart attack. Because of this, following the glycemic load diet is beneficial in better managing diabetes, preventing diabetes complications, driving weight loss in the mid and long-term, and improving your overall health.

Unlike other popular low-carbohydrates, high protein diets, Eating a low Glycemic Load diet has been scientifically proven to help people, as you will see in this chapter:

- control blood sugar and insulin release
- achieve and maintain a healthy weight
- reduce PCOS symptoms
- maintain a healthy condition
- reduce the risk of type 2 diabetes
- improve women's gestational diabetes management and reduce adverse pregnancy outcomes.
- reduce the risk of developing metabolic syndrome dramatically
- prevent heart attack and stroke

LOW-GLYCEMIC LOAD DIET AND INSULIN RESISTANCE REVERSAL

Insulin resistance is a serious and silent health condition that occurs when cells in your muscles, liver, and body fat start ignoring the signal that the insulin hormone is sending out to transfer sugar out of the bloodstream and put it into your body cells. As insulin resistance develops, the body reacts by producing more and more insulin to lower blood sugar.

Over time, the β cells in the pancreas working hard to make a higher supply of insulin can no longer provide more and more insulin. Your blood sugar may reflect the pancreas' inability to maintain the level in the healthy range, and your blood sugar rises, showing pre-diabetes or, at worst, type 2 diabetes.

Insulin resistance is silent and presents no symptoms in its first development stage. The symptoms appear later when the condition worsens, and the pancreas cannot produce enough insulin to maintain your blood glucose within the normal range. When this occurs, the symptoms may be severe, including metabolic syndrome, polycystic ovary syndrome (PCOS), and various types of diabetes.

Fortunately, it is possible to reduce the effects of insulin resistance and boost your insulin sensitivity by following a low-glycemic index diet.

Thus, for many of you, following a low-glycemic diet goes beyond weight-loss management and target the management of particular health condition sensitive to such kind of diet and particularly those related to insulin resistance like:

- excessive hunger
- lethargy or tiredness
- difficulty concentrating
- brain fog
- waist weight gain
- high blood pressure

HIGH-GLYCEMIC INDEX FOODS AFFECT YOUR WEIGHT AND HEALTH.

Consuming high glycemic-load foods may be harmful to your health and causes weight gain because such foods will quickly raise your blood glucose level and cause a blood sugar spike compared to low glycemic foods.

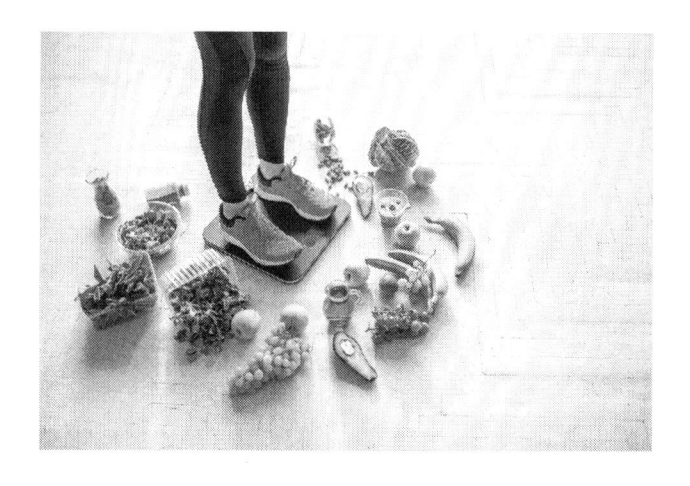

High-glycemic food consumption has also been associated with obesity, insulin resistance, fatty liver, metabolic syndrome, and a higher risk of chronic disease.

WEIGHT GAIN AND HIGH-GLYCEMIC INDEX FOODS

When you eat, food moves to your stomach and intestines, where it is broken down into macronutrients and micronutrients, which are absorbed and transported by your bloodstream. The pancreas produces insulin through its beta cells. It releases it into the bloodstream when we eat to allow body cells, including muscles and other cells, to absorb and transform sugar (glucose) into energy throughout the body.

Insulin also sends signals to the liver, muscle, and adipocytes (fat cells) to store the excess glucose for further use:

- in muscle tissues as glycogen.
- in the liver as glycogen.
- in adipose tissue (fat reserves of the body) in the form of triglycerides, which are fat molecules that store energy

LOW-GLYCEMIC LOAD DIET IS BETTER FOR YOUR BODY

Carbohydrates found in natural foods, such as legumes, fruits, vegetables, meats, fish, and grains, tend to be more complex and harder to digest, translating by a low-glycemic index. Eating such foods will lead to smooth increases and falls in your blood glucose levels, which help sustain your healthy condition, promote weight loss, prevent obesity, and helps diabetes control.

Many studies have also shown the health benefits of selecting foods with a low-glycemic index. Following a low glycemic diet may provide several health benefits, including:

- diabetes management (gestational diabetes, type 1 and type 2 diabetes)
- long-lasting weight loss,
- obesity control,
- reduction of heart strokes
- prevention of coronary heart disease
- PCOS prevention

LOW-GLYCEMIC DIET LOAD LEADS TO HUNGER-REDUCTION

Leptin, referred to as the starvation or "hunger hormone," is a hormone produced by fat tissues and is secreted into our bloodstream. It plays a crucial role in weight regulation by reducing a person's appetite.

Eating low-glycemic-index foods translates to eating a diet that lowers the insulin response and increases circulating leptin levels inducing a post-meal condition favorable for reduced food consumption due to a lower person's appetite. This may be very beneficial in such situations:

- type 2 diabetes management
- obesity control
- weight loss
- weight maintenance management
- insulin resistance

When you eat an adequate combination of foods, you will notice that your appetite is under control due to the leptin effect. Your insulin levels will also stabilize, and your sugar levels will rise and fall smoothly. The consequence will be beneficial since eating less often will lead to weight loss and a healthy lifestyle.

PART IV
ADHERING TO THE GLYCEMIC LOAD DIET RULES

❄

EATING WHOLE AND MINIMALLY PROCESSED FOODS

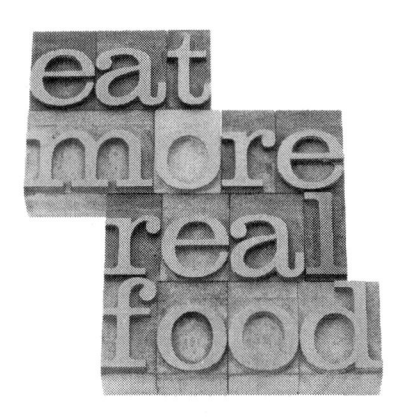

Highly-processed foods are generally industrially-made and contain many ingredients, including high-fructose corn syrup, trans fats, monosodium glutamate, artificial sweeteners, flavors, colors, and other chemical additives. They are believed to be a significant contributor to the obesity epidemic in the world, promoting diabetes, chronic inflammation, and the prevalence of autoimmune diseases. Therefore, you must identify healthy foods to include in your diet and those to exclude because they are considered unhealthy and pro-inflammatory.

Whole foods are unprocessed or minimally processed— natural foods without added sugars, fat, sodium, flavorings, or other artificial ingredients. Whole foods have little to no additives or preservatives. They are generally close to their natural state, unprocessed, and unrefined.

Whole foods and minimally processed foods are generally low to moderate in calories and high in fiber and nutrients. Most vegetables, fruits, beans, meats, poultry, fish, dairy products, and nuts are low glycemic in their raw state.

The glycemic load diet includes a variety of healthy foods loaded with high-quality carbohydrates, fats, proteins, vitamins, and minerals. This includes:

- dark-green vegetables
- red & orange vegetables
- beans, peas, lentils
- non-starchy vegetables
- starchy Vegetables
- fruits
- grains
- dairy and alternatives
- meats (lean or low-fat)
- seafood
- nuts, seeds, soy products

The serving sizes of different foods are provided in part V, "meal planning guidelines."

EATING LOW GLYCEMIC AND ANTI-INFLAMMATORY FOODS

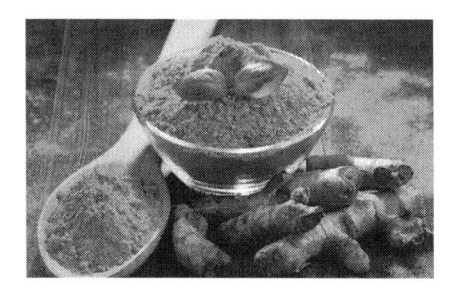

EATING LOW GLYCEMIC LOAD VEGETABLES AND FRUITS

Vegetables and fruits constitute an essential part of a diabetes-friendly diet. A diet rich in low glycemic load vegetables and fruits positively affects your blood sugar and blood pressure. In addition, non-starchy vegetables and fruits are good sources of anti-inflammatory nutrients such as polyphenols, antioxidants, and flavonoids which contribute to lowering inflammation and, in turn, reducing the risk of diabetes complications.

The serving sizes for low glycemic load vegetables and fruits are equivalent to (please refer to part V for more details)

- 1 cup raw or salad vegetables
- ½ cup cooked vegetables
- ¾ cup (6oz) vegetable juice homemade and unsweetened
- • ½ cup of cooked beans, lentils, and peas
- • 1 medium piece of fruit
- • 1 cup (6 oz) of sliced fruits
- • ½ cup (4 oz) of fruit juice

The total vegetable intake (per day) is equivalent to 8-10 servings. You have to vary your meals using the maximal recommended amount as follows:

• "Dark-Green Vegetables" group up to 2 servings

• "Red & Orange Vegetables" group up to 3 servings

• "Beans, Peas, Lentils" group up to 2 servings

• "Starchy Vegetables" group up to 1 serving

• "Other Vegetables" group up to 3 servings

The total fruit intake is equivalent to 2-4 servings per day.

Choosing healthy fats

The glycemic load diet is rich in omega-3 and low in omega-6 than most diets. High levels of omega-3 combined with a low (omega-6/omega-3) are associated with many health benefits, including a significant reduction of unnecessary inflammation and diabetes complications. For example, a ratio (omega-6/omega-3) of 4/1 was correlated to a 70% reduction in mortality. So, based on recent studies, you have to keep the ratio (omega-6/omega-3) in the range of 1/1 and 4/1, which is associated with positive health outcomes.

Strategies to achieve an adequate ratio (omega-6/omega-3) include

- consuming fatty fish (e.g., sardines, mackerels, salmon, herring, anchovies) twice a week,
- consuming nuts and seeds (e.g., flax seeds, chia seeds, walnuts) twice a week.

INCREASING OLIVE OIL CONSUMPTION

Recent studies have established that an extra virgin olive oil-rich diet reduces blood glucose levels, LDL cholesterol (bad), and triglycerides. In addition, extra virgin olive oil was found to provide potential benefits for weight loss, diabetes prevention, and management.

The anti-diabetes benefits of Extra Virgin Olive Oil (EVOO) increase with the daily ingested amount. A minimum of extra virgin olive oil of four tablespoons per day is necessary to provide beneficial anti-diabetes and antioxidant effects. When cooking, EVOO is an excellent choice as it has been well established that it helps reduce blood sugar levels, reduce blood pressure, lower bad cholesterol (LDL), and decrease inflammation. The nutritional composition of virgin olive is comprised mainly of:

- monounsaturated fatty acids (69.2% for extra virgin olive oil), mainly Oleic acid (omega-9)
- saturated fats (15.4% for extra virgin olive oil), mainly Stearic acid and Palmitic Acid
- polyunsaturated (9.07% for extra virgin olive oil), mainly Linoleic acid (omega-3)
- polyphenols
- vitamin E, carotenoids, and squalene

Strategies to increase your daily intake of olive oil include

- replacing butter with EVOO,

- using olive oil as finishing oil for your meals,
- replacing the oil you use for cooking,
- roasting, and frying with EVOO.

INCLUDING ANTI-INFLAMMATORY SPICES IN YOUR DIET

Over the last decades, extensive research has revealed that some spices and their active components exhibit tremendous anti-inflammatory benefits. Thus, herbs have been found to prevent or decrease the severity of diabetes complications and several chronic conditions such as arthritis, asthma, multiple sclerosis, cardiovascular diseases, lupus, cancer, and neurodegenerative diseases. The most common spices used for their anti-inflammatory activities are

- turmeric,
- green tea,
- garlic,
- ginger,
- cayenne pepper,
- black pepper,
- black cumin,
- clove,
- cumin,
- ginseng,
- cardamom,
- parsley
- cinnamon,
- rosemary,
- chives,
- basil,
- cilantro

In addition, spices have the unique property of adding flavor to any meal without adding fats or salt. Therefore, you should consider integrating herbs into your daily diet when cooking.

Some strategies for getting more herbs and spices in your diet include

- using some fresh herbs as the main ingredient (e.g., herb salad, tabbouleh salad),
- replacing some green vegetables in salads with herbs,
- substituting (or reducing) salt in a recipe with spices,
- replacing mayonnaise with basil-olive oil preparation,
- drinking 3–4 cups of green tea daily.

Drinking more water

Water is critical for life. Without water, there is no life. All of the organs of our body, such as the heart, brain, lungs, and muscles, contain a significant quantity of water and need water to stay healthy.

Every day we lose water, and we need to replace it through a regular water supply. Otherwise, we can suffer from dehydration, which may alter the normal body's functions.

The recommended water intake for men aged 19+ is 3 liters (13 cups), and for women aged 19+ is 2.2 liters (9 cups) each day.

AVOIDING HIGH GLYCEMIC AND INFLAMMATORY FOODS

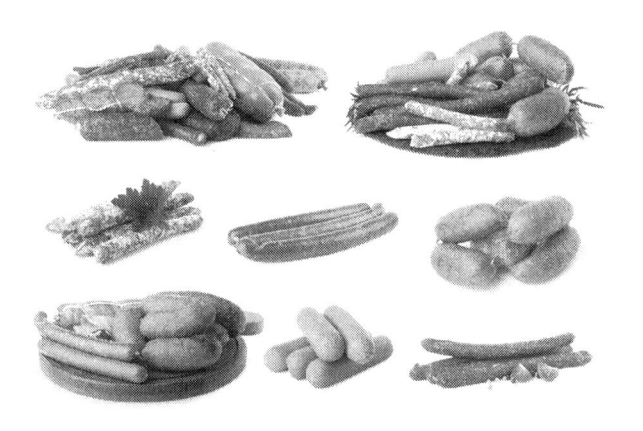

LIMITING MODERATE GLYCEMIC FOODS AND AVOIDING HIGH GLYCEMIC FOODS

People with diabetes must pay attention to the glycemic load of foods to prevent eating high amounts of glucose and experiencing abrupt spikes in blood sugar.

For a standard serving size of food, glycemic load (GL) is considered high with GL greater or equal to 20, medium with GL in the range of 11-19, and low with GL less or equal to 10.

You should then eat foods with GL under or equal to 10, and keep in mind that your daily allowance of GL must not exceed 50 (in a 2000-calorie diet)

Excluding Trans-Fats containing Foods

Trans-fatty acids are mostly industrially manufactured fats made during the hydrogenation process. Trans fats provide foods with a desirable taste and texture. However, unlike other dietary fats, consuming trans-fatty acids raises your bad cholesterol (LDL), lowers your good cholesterol (HDL) levels, increases your risk of developing severe cardiovascular conditions, and aggravates inflammation. Trans fats may be present in several food products, including:

- fried fast foods (i.e., french fries, fried chicken, battered fish, mozzarella sticks, and doughnuts)
- margarine
- peanut butter
- baked goods (i.e., cakes, cookies, and pies made with margarine or vegetable shortening)
- vegetable shortening

Strategies to reduce drastically trans fats intake include

- avoiding or reducing intake of fried fast foods—including french fries, fried chicken, battered fish, mozzarella sticks, doughnuts, margarine, peanut butter, frozen pizza, baked goods made with margarine or vegetable shortening
- eating smaller portion sizes
- consuming trans-fat-containing foods less frequently.

EATING A LITTLE LESS RED MEAT BUT ENOUGH PROTEINS

There is little evidence that red meat may contribute to inflammation and alter glycemic control. At the same time, some recent studies revealed that unprocessed red meats might be associated with less inflammation and are safe for people with diabetes or pre-diabetes. However, there is a consensus about the danger of consuming processed red meat such as sausage, bacon, salami, and hot dogs. A 2012 study funded and supported by some health and nutrition government agencies has established the link between processed red meal consumption and increased total mortality. The study revealed that replacing one serving of red meat daily with other protein sources such as fish, poultry, and nuts could decrease mortality risk by 7-19%. It also revealed that daily unprocessed red meat consumption raised mortality risk by 13%.

These findings suggest restricting your red meat intake reduces inflammation and prevents diabetes complications.

Eating adequate protein amounts is extremely important for your health because proteins play a crucial role in your body's vital processes and metabolisms. The weekly recommended proteins intake is equivalent to:

- 30 servings of animal proteins (mainly lean white meat and eggs)
- 10 servings of seafood
- 5 servings of nuts and seeds

By restricting red meat intake in the range of 1/5 to 1/4 of animal proteins (e.g., 6 to 7.5 servings of red meat per week), you may experience improvement in your overall health and reduction of some symptoms caused by inflammation.

PART V
MEAL PLANNING GUIDELINES

MEAL PLANNING GUIDELINES

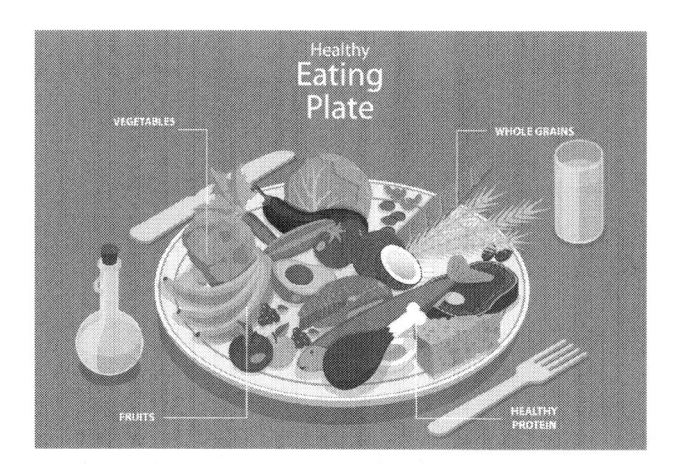

Meal planning allows you to make making informed choices that will promote weight loss and optimal health. Instead of giving strict recommendations, it gives you options for each food group you can choose.

All foods are assumed to be:

- low glycemic load
- unprocessed or minimally processed
- in nutrient-dense forms
- lean or low-fat
- prepared and cooked with minimal added sugars, salt (sodium), refined carbohydrates, saturated fat, or trans fats.

The total daily calories depend on your personal needs. You have to follow the general guidelines in the next chapters. Recommended amounts of foods in each food group are given to allow you to design your weekly and monthly eating plan.

The five categories of foods are:

- vegetables
- fruits
- grains
- dairy and fortified soy alternatives
- protein foods

VEGETABLES AND VEGETABLES PRODUCTS

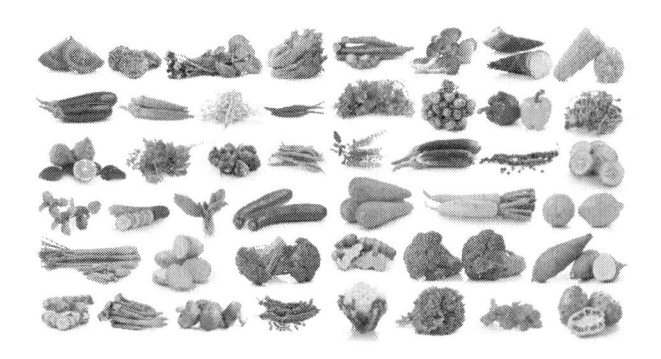

■ WHAT IS THE PORTION SIZE?

The typical serving sizes for vegetables and vegetable juices are equivalent to:

- 1 cup raw or salad vegetables
- ½ cup cooked vegetables
- ¾ cup (6 oz) vegetable juice homemade and unsweetened
- ½ cup of cooked beans, lentils, and peas

All vegetables in this list have low glycemic load values.

◼ How Much a Day?

Total vegetable intake: up to 10 servings

- "Dark-Green Vegetables" group up to 2 servings
- "Red & Orange Vegetables" group up to 3 servings
- "Beans, Peas, Lentils" group up to 2 servings
- "Starchy Vegetables" group up to 3 servings
- "Other Vegetables" group up to 3 servings

For most people, following the glycemic load diet will require an increase in total vegetable intake from all five vegetable subgroups ("Dark-Green Vegetables", "Red & Orange Vegetables", "Beans, Peas, Lentils", "Starchy Vegetables", "Other Vegetables").

Strategies to increase total vegetable intake include

1. increasing the vegetable content of mixed dishes (more vegetables)
2. adding vegetables to breakfast
3. blending and consuming vegetables into smoothies
4. preparing sauces with vegetables
5. consuming regularly vegetable-based soups

◼ DARK-GREEN VEGETABLES: THE SIMPLIFIED LIST

- **amaranth leaves** (all fresh, frozen, cooked, or raw)
- **arugula (rocket)** (all fresh, frozen, cooked, or raw)
- **bok choy (Chinese chard)** (all fresh, frozen, cooked, or raw)

- **bitter melon leaves** (all fresh, frozen, cooked, or raw)
- **broccoli** (all fresh, frozen, cooked, or raw)
- **chamnamul** (all fresh, frozen, cooked, or raw)
- **chard (all fresh, frozen, cooked, or raw)**
- **collards** (all fresh, frozen, cooked, or raw)
- **dandelion greens** (all fresh, frozen, cooked, or raw)
- **endive** (all fresh, frozen, cooked, or raw)
- **escarole** (all fresh, frozen, cooked, or raw)
- **kale** (all fresh, frozen, cooked, or raw)
- **mixed greens** (all fresh, frozen, cooked, or raw)
- **mustard greens** (all fresh, frozen, cooked, or raw)
- **poke greens** (all fresh, frozen, cooked, or raw)
- **rapini** (all fresh, frozen, cooked, or raw)
- **romaine lettuce** (all fresh, frozen, cooked, or raw)
- **spinach (all fresh, frozen, cooked, or raw)**
- **swiss chard** (all fresh, frozen, cooked, or raw)
- **taro leaves (all fresh, frozen, cooked, or raw)**
- **turnip greens** (all fresh, frozen, cooked, or raw)
- **watercress** (all fresh, frozen, cooked, or raw)

■ RED AND ORANGE VEGETABLES: THE SIMPLIFIED LIST

- **acorn squash** (all fresh, frozen, vegetables or juice, cooked or raw)
- **butternut squash** (all fresh, frozen, vegetables or juice, cooked or raw)
- **calabaza** (all fresh, frozen, vegetables or juice, cooked or raw)
- **carrots** (all fresh, frozen, vegetables or juice, cooked or raw)
- **red bell peppers** (all fresh, frozen, vegetables or juice, cooked or raw)

- **hubbard squash** (all fresh, frozen, vegetables or juice, cooked or raw)
- **orange bell peppers** (all fresh, frozen, vegetables or juice, cooked or raw)
- **sweet potatoes** (all fresh, frozen, vegetables or juice, cooked or raw)
- **tomatoes** (all fresh, frozen, vegetables or juice, cooked or raw)
- **pumpkin** (all fresh, frozen, vegetables or juice, cooked or raw)
- **winter squash** (all fresh, frozen, vegetables or juice, cooked or raw)

■ BEANS, PEAS, LENTILS: THE SIMPLIFIED LIST

- **beans** (all cooked from dry)
- **peas** (all cooked from dry)
- **chickpeas (Garbanzo Beans)** (all cooked from dry)
- **lentils** (all cooked from dry)
- **black beans** (all cooked from dry)
- **black-eyed peas** (all cooked from dry)
- **Bayo beans** (all cooked from dry)
- **cannellini beans** (all cooked from dry)
- **great northern beans** (all cooked from dry)
- **edamame** (all cooked from dry)
- **kidney beans** (all cooked from dry)
- **lentils** (all cooked from dry)
- **lima beans** (all cooked from dry)
- **mung beans** (all cooked from dry)
- **pigeon peas** (all cooked from dry)
- **pinto beans** (all cooked from dry)
- **split peas** (all cooked from dry)

■ Starchy Vegetables: The Simplified List

- **breadfruit** (all fresh, or frozen)
- **burdock root** (all fresh, or frozen)
- **cassava** (all fresh, or frozen)
- **jicama** (all fresh, or frozen)
- **lotus root** (all fresh, or frozen)
- **plantains** (all fresh, or frozen)
- **salsify** (all fresh, or frozen)
- **taro root (dasheen or yautia)** (all fresh, or frozen)
- **water chestnuts** (all fresh, or frozen)
- **yam** (all fresh, or frozen)
- **yucca** (all fresh, or frozen)

■ OTHER VEGETABLES: THE SIMPLIFIED LIST

- **asparagus** (all fresh, frozen, cooked, or raw)
- **avocado** (all fresh, frozen, cooked, or raw)
- **bamboo shoots** (all fresh, frozen, cooked, or raw)
- **beets** (all fresh, frozen, cooked, or raw)
- **bitter melon** (all fresh, frozen, cooked, or raw)
- **Brussels sprouts** (all fresh, frozen, cooked, or raw)
- **green cabbage** (all fresh, frozen, cooked, or raw)
- **savoy cabbage** (all fresh, frozen, cooked, or raw)
- **red cabbage** (all fresh, frozen, cooked, or raw)
- **cactus pads** (all fresh, frozen, cooked, or raw)
- **cauliflower** (all fresh, frozen, cooked, or raw)
- **celery** (all fresh, frozen, cooked, or raw)
- **chayote (mirliton)** (all fresh, frozen, cooked, or raw)
- **cucumber** (all fresh, frozen, cooked, or raw)
- **eggplant** (all fresh, frozen, cooked, or raw)
- **green beans** (all fresh, frozen, cooked, or raw)

- **kohlrabi** (all fresh, frozen, cooked, or raw)
- **luffa** (all fresh, frozen, cooked, or raw)
- **mushrooms** (all fresh, frozen, cooked, or raw)
- **okra** (all fresh, frozen, cooked, or raw)
- **onions** (all fresh, frozen, cooked, or raw)
- **radish** (all fresh, frozen, cooked, or raw)
- **rutabaga** (all fresh, frozen, cooked, or raw)
- **seaweed** (all fresh, frozen, cooked, or raw)
- **snow peas** (all fresh, frozen, cooked, or raw)
- **summer squash** (all fresh, frozen, cooked, or raw)
- **tomatillos** (all fresh, frozen, cooked, or raw)

FRUITS AND FRUITS PRODUCTS

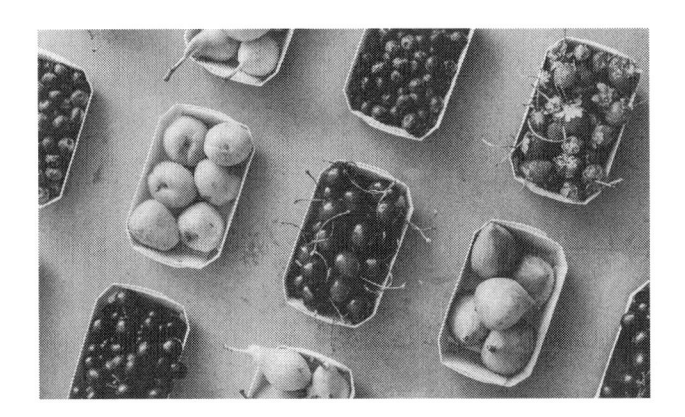

Having diabetes does not imply you can't eat fruit. Instead, you'll choose low glycemic load fruits. The majority of fruit and vegetables are nutrient-dense, low-calorie, and packed full of essential nutrients such as vitamins, minerals, and fiber.

■ WHAT IS THE PORTION SIZE?

The typical serving sizes for fruits and fruits juices are equivalent to:

- 1 medium piece
- 1 cup (6 oz) of sliced fruits
- ¾ cup (6 oz) of fruit juice

How Much a Day?

2 to 4 servings per day

The fruit food group comprises whole fruits and fruit products (100% fruit juice). Whole fruits can be eaten in various forms, such as cut, cubed, sliced, or diced. At least 60% of the recommended amount of total fruit should come from whole fruit rather than 100% juice. Juices should be without added sugars or food additives.

For most people, following the low-glycemic diet will require increasing the total fruit. Strategies to increase total fruit intake include

1. often consuming fruits
2. adding fruits to breakfast.
3. choosing more whole fruits as snacks
4. blending and consuming fruits into smoothies
5. choosing and carrying fruit with you to eat later
6. creating adequate pairings with your favorite foods

■ FRUITS: THE SIMPLIFIED LIST

- **apples** (all fresh, frozen, dried fruits or 100% fruit juices)
- **Asian pears** (all fresh, frozen, dried fruits or 100% fruit juices)
- **bananas** (all fresh, frozen, dried fruits or 100% fruit juices)

- **blackberries** (all fresh, frozen, dried fruits or 100% fruit juices)
- **blueberries** (all fresh, frozen, dried fruits or 100% fruit juices)
- **currants** (all fresh, frozen, dried fruits or 100% fruit juices)
- **huckleberries** (all fresh, frozen, dried fruits or 100% fruit juices)
- **kiwifruit** (all fresh, frozen, dried fruits or 100% fruit juices)
- **mulberries** (all fresh, frozen, dried fruits or 100% fruit juices)
- **raspberries** (all fresh, frozen, dried fruits or 100% fruit juices)
- **strawberries** (all fresh, frozen, dried fruits or 100% fruit juices)
- **calamondin** (all fresh, frozen, dried fruits or 100% fruit juices)
- **grapefruit** (all fresh, frozen, dried fruits or 100% fruit juices)
- **lemons** (all fresh, frozen, dried fruits or 100% fruit juices)
- **limes** (all fresh, frozen, dried fruits or 100% fruit juices)
- **oranges** (all fresh, frozen, dried fruits or 100% fruit juices)
- **pomelos** (all fresh, frozen, dried fruits or 100% fruit juices)
- **cherries** (all fresh, frozen, dried fruits or 100% fruit juices)
- **dates** (all fresh, frozen, dried fruits or 100% fruit juices)
- **figs** (all fresh, frozen, dried fruits or 100% fruit juices)
- **grapes** (all fresh, frozen, dried fruits or 100% fruit juices)
- **guava** (all fresh, frozen, dried fruits or 100% fruit juices)
- **lychee** (all fresh, frozen, dried fruits or 100% fruit juices)
- **mangoes** (all fresh, frozen, dried fruits or 100% fruit juices)
- **nectarines** (all fresh, frozen, dried fruits or 100% fruit juices)
- **peaches** (all fresh, frozen, dried fruits or 100% fruit juices)
- **pears** (all fresh, frozen, dried fruits or 100% fruit juices)
- **plums** (all fresh, frozen, dried fruits or 100% fruit juices)
- **pomegranates** (all fresh, frozen, dried fruits or 100% fruit juices)
- **rhubarb** (all fresh, frozen, dried fruits or 100% fruit juices)
- **sapote** (all fresh, frozen, dried fruits or 100% fruit juices)
- **soursop** (all fresh, frozen, dried fruits or 100% fruit juices)

GRAINS

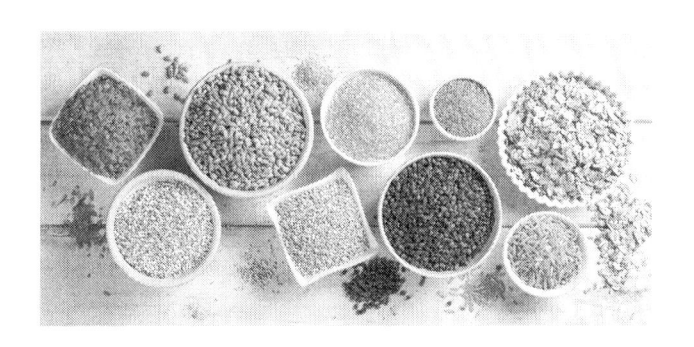

■ WHAT IS THE PORTION SIZE?

The typical serving sizes for cereals and grains are equivalent to:

- ⅓ cup breakfast cereal or muesli
- ½ cup of cooked cereal, or other cooked grain
- ⅓ cup of cooked rice (white rice excluded), and other small grains
- ½ cup of cold cereal

How Much a Day?

Up to 3 servings per day.

■ WHOLE GRAINS: THE SIMPLIFIED LIST

- **barley** (all whole-grain products or used as ingredients)
- **brown rice** (all whole-grain products or used as ingredients)
- **buckwheat** (all whole-grain products or used as ingredients)
- **bulgur** (all whole-grain products or used as ingredients)
- **millet** (all whole-grain products or used as ingredients)
- **oats (Avena sativa L.)** (all whole-grain products or used as ingredients)
- **quinoa** (all whole-grain products or used as ingredients)
- **dark rye** (all whole-grain products or used as ingredients)
- **whole-wheat bread** (all whole-grain products or used as ingredients)
- **whole-wheat chapati** (all whole-grain products or used as ingredients)
- **whole-grain cereals** (all whole-grain products or used as ingredients)
- **wild rice** (all whole-grain products or used as ingredients)

DAIRY AND FORTIFIED SOY ALTERNATIVES

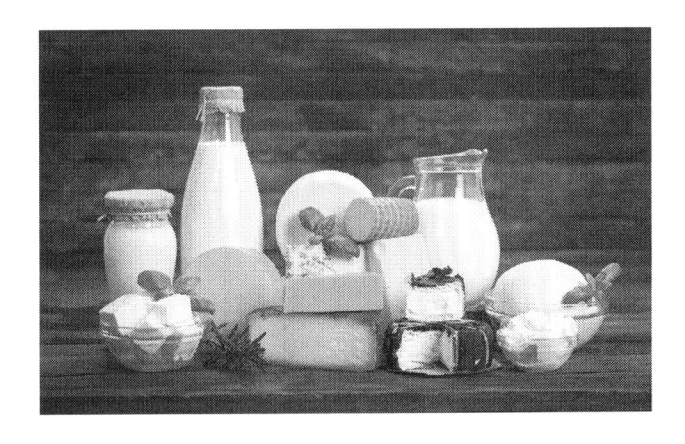

■ WHAT IS THE PORTION SIZE?

The typical serving sizes for dairy products are equivalent to:

- 1 cup of milk, soy beverage, or yogurt
- ⅓ cup of cottage cheese
- 1 oz of cheese

People with celiac disease or lactose intolerance should consume dairy alternatives

How Much a Day?

Up to 3 servings per day

■ DAIRY AND FORTIFIED SOY ALTERNATIVES: THE SIMPLIFIED LIST

- **buttermilk** (all fluid, evaporated milk, or dry including lactose-free and lactose-reduced products)
- **soy beverages** (all fluid, evaporated milk, or dry including lactose-free and lactose-reduced products)
- **soy milk** (all fluid, evaporated milk, or dry including lactose-free and lactose-reduced products)
- **yogurt** (without added sugar and food additives) (all fluid, evaporated milk, or dry including lactose-free and lactose-reduced products)
- **kefir** (without added sugar and food additives) (all fluid, evaporated milk, or dry including lactose-free and lactose-reduced products)
- **frozen yogurt** (without added sugar and food additives) (all fluid, evaporated milk, or dry including lactose-free and lactose-reduced products)
- **cheeses** (all fluid, evaporated milk, or dry including lactose-free and lactose-reduced products)

PROTEIN FOODS

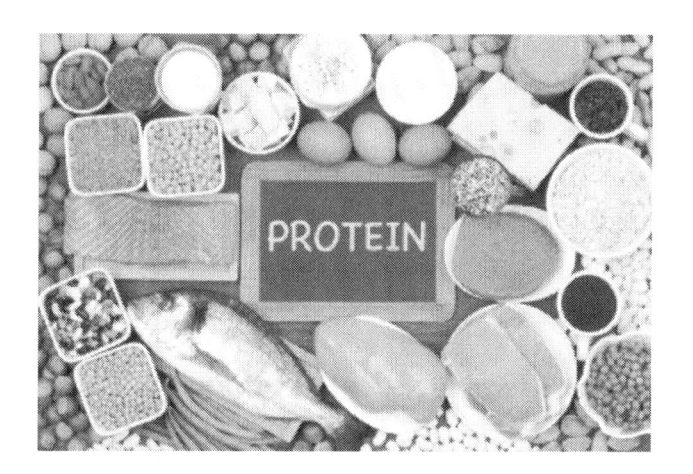

❄

Eating a daily adequate amount of protein is very important for your health. Unlike carbohydrates and fat, your body does not store protein, and you need to eat enough to stay healthy. Animal-based foods are excellent protein sources because they offer a complete composition of essential amino acids with higher bioavailability and digestibility (>90%). Therefore, the main principle to observe here when designing your meal program is to keep a weekly proteins intake equivalent to:

- 30 servings of animal proteins (mainly lean white meat and eggs)
- 10 servings of seafood
- 5 servings of nuts and seeds

■ MEATS, POULTRY, EGGS, SEAFOODS: WHAT IS THE PORTION SIZE?

The typical serving sizes for the "meats, poultry, eggs", "seafood", and "nuts, seeds, soy Products" groups are equivalent to:

- 3 to 4 ounces of cooked, baked, or broiled beef
- 3 to 4 ounces of cooked, baked, or broiled veal
- 3 to 4 ounces of cooked, baked, or broiled poultry
- 3 to 4 ounces of cooked or canned fish
- 3 to 4 ounces of seafood
- 2 medium eggs
- ⅓ cup of nuts (5 large or 10 small nuts)
- 2 tablespoons of nut butter
- 2 tablespoons of nut spread

■ Meats, Poultry, Eggs: The simplified List

Meats (lean or low-fats) include:

- beef, goat, lamb, and pork (fat red meats must be limited due to their pro-inflammatory effects). You have to choose lean meats preferably grass-fed beef, lamb, or bison
- game meat (e.g., bison, moose, elk, deer)

Poultry (lean or low-fats) includes

- chicken

- turkey
- cornish hens
- duck
- game birds (e.g., ostrich, pheasant, and quail)
- goose.

Eggs include

- chicken eggs
- turkey eggs
- duck eggs and other birds' eggs

■ Seafood: The simplified List

Seafood include

- salmon
- sardine
- anchovy
- black sea bass
- catfish
- clams
- cod
- crab
- crawfish
- flounder
- haddock
- hake
- herring
- lobster
- mullet
- oyster
- perch

- pollock
- scallop
- shrimp
- sole
- squid
- tilapia
- freshwater trout
- tuna

■ NUTS, SEEDS, SOY PRODUCTS: THE SIMPLIFIED LIST

Nuts (and nut butter) include

- almonds
- pecans
- Brazil nuts
- pistachios
- hazelnuts
- macadamias
- pine nuts
- walnuts
- cashew nuts

Seeds (and seed butter) include:

- pumpkin seeds
- psyllium seeds
- chia seeds.
- flax seeds
- sunflower seeds
- sesame seeds
- poppy seeds

PART VI
THE BEST FOODS (LOW GLYCEMIC LOAD FOODS)

BAKED PRODUCTS

Apple Strudel ☛ Serving size= 1 oz, 28.4 g; GI= 59 (Medium); GL= 6.5 (Low); Net carb= 11 g

Bagel Multigrain ☛ Serving size= 1 miniature, 26 g; GI= 43 (Low); GL= 5 (Low); Net carb= 11.6 g

Bagel Multigrain With Raisins ☛ Serving size= 1 miniature, 26 g; GI= 49 (Low); GL= 6.1 (Low); Net carb= 12.4 g

Bagel Oat Bran ☛ Serving size= 1 miniature, 26 g; GI= 47 (Low); GL= 5.5 (Low); Net carb= 11.6 g

Bagel Pumpernickel ☛ Serving size= 1 miniature, 26 g; GI= 50 (Low); GL= 5.8 (Low); Net carb= 11.6 g

Bagel Wheat ☛ Serving size= 1 miniature, 26 g; GI= 71 (High); GL= 8.2 (Low); Net carb= 11.6 g

Bagel Wheat Bran ☛ Serving size= 1 miniature, 26 g; GI= 65 (Medium); GL= 7.5 (Low); Net carb= 11.6 g

Bagel Whole Grain White ☛ Serving size= 1 miniature, 26 g; GI= 72 (High); GL= 8.4 (Low); Net carb= 11.6 g

Bagel Whole Wheat ☛ Serving size= 1 miniature, 26 g; GI= 71 (High); GL= 8.2 (Low); Net carb= 11.6 g

Bagel, white ☛ Serving size= 1 miniature, 26 g; GI= 72 (High); GL= 9.5 (Low); Net carb= 13.2 g

Biscuit, Cheese ☛ Serving size= 1 biscuit (2 inch dia), 30 g; GI= 70 (High); GL= 9.8 (Low); Net carb= 14 g

Biscuit, Mixed Grain Refrigerated Dough ☛ Serving size= 1 oz, 28.4 g; GI= 70 (High); GL= 9.5 (Low); Net carb= 13.5 g

Biscuit, Plain Or Buttermilk Made From Recipe ☛ Serving size= 1 oz, 28.4 g; GI= 70 (High); GL= 8.5 (Low); Net carb= 12.2 g

Biscuit, Whole Wheat ☛ Serving size= 1 small (1-1/2 inch dia), 14 g; GI= 70 (High); GL= 3.9 (Low); Net carb= 5.5 g

Bread, 100% Whole Grain ☛ Serving size= 1 slice, 1 oz, 28.4 g; GI= 53 (Low); GL= 5.9 (Low); Net carb= 11.2 g

Bread, Barley ☛ Serving size= 1 slice, 1 oz, 28.4 g; GI= 68 (Medium); GL= 8.5 (Low); Net carb= 12.5 g

Bread, Buckwheat ☛ Serving size= 1 slice, 1 oz, 28.4 g; GI= 47 (Low); GL= 6.2 (Low); Net carb= 13.2 g

Bread, Cinnamon ☛ Serving size= 1 slice, 1 oz, 28.4 g; GI= 72 (High); GL= 8.4 (Low); Net carb= 11.6 g

Bread, CornBread, Made From Recipe Made ☛ Serving size= 1 slice, 1 oz, 28.4 g; GI= 75 (High); GL= 9.3 (Low); Net carb= 12.4 g

Bread, Cracked-Wheat ☛ Serving size= 1 slice, 1 oz, 28.4 g; GI= 73 (High); GL= 9.1 (Low); Net carb= 12.5 g

Bread, Dough Fried ☛ Serving size= 1 slice or roll, 26 g; GI= 66 (Medium); GL= 7.5 (Low); Net carb= 11.3 g

Bread, Gluten-free multigrain ☛ Serving size= 1 slice, 1 oz, 28.4 g; GI= 73 (High); GL= 8.6 (Low); Net carb= 11.8 g

Bread, Italian ☛ Serving size= 1 oz, 28.4 g; GI= 70 (High); GL= 9.2 (Low); Net carb= 13.1 g

Bread, Linseed Rye ☛ Serving size= 1 slice, 1 oz, 28.4 g; GI= 55 (Medium); GL= 4.7 (Low); Net carb= 8.5 g

Bread, Pita ☛ Serving size= 1 slice, 1 oz, 28.4 g; GI= 57 (Medium); GL= 8.7 (Low); Net carb= 15.2 g

Bread, Rice Bran ☛ Serving size= 1 oz, 28.4 g; GI= 66 (Medium); GL= 7.3 (Low); Net carb= 11 g

Bread, Rye ☛ Serving size= 1 slice, 1 oz, 28.4 g; GI= 59 (Medium); GL= 7.8 (Low); Net carb= 13.2 g

Bread, Soy ☛ Serving size= 1 oz, 28.4 g; GI= 44 (Low); GL= 4.7 (Low); Net carb= 10.7 g

Bread, Sunflower And Barley ☛ Serving size= 1 slice, 1 oz, 28.4 g; GI= 57 (Medium); GL= 5.2 (Low); Net carb= 9.2 g

Bread, Wholegrain pumpernickel ☛ Serving size= 1 slice, 1 oz, 28.4 g; GI= 46 (Low); GL= 3.3 (Low); Net carb= 7.2 g

Butter Croissants ☛ Serving size= 1 oz, 28.4 g; GI= 71 (High); GL= 8.7 (Low); Net carb= 12.3 g

Cake, Chocolate Fudge Cherry ☛ Serving size= 1 oz, 28.4 g; GI= 55 (Medium); GL= 5.9 (Low); Net carb= 10.7 g

Cake, Sponge Made From Recipe ☛ Serving size= 1 oz, 28.4 g; GI= 55 (Medium); GL= 9 (Low); Net carb= 16.4 g

Churros ☛ Serving size= 1 churro, 26 g; GI= 66 (Medium); GL= 8.4 (Low); Net carb= 12.7 g

Coconut Custard Pie ☛ Serving size= 1 oz, 28.4 g; GI= 53 (Low); GL= 4.3 (Low); Net carb= 8.1 g

Coookie, Butter With Fruit And/or Nuts ☛ Serving size= 1 miniature/bite size, 5 g; GI= 69 (Medium); GL= 2.2 (Low); Net carb= 3.2 g

Corn Flour Patty Or Tart Fried ☛ Serving size= 1 patty, 10 g; GI= 75 (High); GL= 2.9 (Low); Net carb= 3.8 g

CornBread, Made From Home Recipe ☛ Serving size= 1 surface inch, 11 g; GI= 75 (High); GL= 3.4 (Low); Net carb= 4.5 g

Cornmeal, Fritter Puerto Rican Style ☛ Serving size= 1 fritter, 40 g; GI= 71 (High); GL= 5.6 (Low); Net carb= 7.9 g

Cornmeal, Stick Puerto Rican Style ☛ Serving size= 1 stick, 20 g; GI= 75 (High); GL= 6.9 (Low); Net carb= 9.2 g

Crackers, Cheese Regular ☛ Serving size= 1/2 oz, 14.2 g; GI= 67 (Medium); GL= 5.4 (Low); Net carb= 8.1 g

Crackers, Water Biscuits ☛ Serving size= 4 cracker 1 serving, 14 g; GI= 69 (Medium); GL= 6.3 (Low); Net carb= 9.2 g

Crackers, Wheat ☛ Serving size= 1/2 oz, 14.2 g; GI= 71 (High); GL= 6.1 (Low); Net carb= 8.6 g

Crackers, Whole-Wheat ☛ Serving size= 1/2 oz, 14.2 g; GI= 66 (Medium); GL= 5.5 (Low); Net carb= 8.3 g

Cream Puff Shell Made From Recipe ☛ Serving size= 1 oz, 28.4 g; GI= 55 (Medium); GL= 3.4 (Low); Net carb= 6.2 g

Croissant Chocolate ☛ Serving size= 1 oz, 28.4 g; GI= 73 (High); GL= 9.6 (Low); Net carb= 13.1 g

Croissant Fruit ☛ Serving size= 1 oz, 28.4 g; GI= 71 (High); GL= 8.9 (Low); Net carb= 12.5 g

Croissants Apple ☛ Serving size= 1 oz, 28.4 g; GI= 71 (High); GL= 7 (Low); Net carb= 9.8 g

Croutons Seasoned ☛ Serving size= 1/2 oz, 14.2 g; GI= 70 (High); GL= 5.8 (Low); Net carb= 8.3 g

Crumpet ☛ Serving size= 1 small (2-1/2 inch dia), 20 g; GI= 73 (High); GL= 3.9 (Low); Net carb= 5.3 g

Danish Pastry, Cheese ☛ Serving size= 1 oz, 28.4 g; GI= 63 (Medium); GL= 6.5 (Low); Net carb= 10.3 g

Danish Pastry, Cinnamon ☛ Serving size= 1 oz, 28.4 g; GI= 63 (Medium); GL= 7.7 (Low); Net carb= 12.3 g

Danish Pastry, with Fruit (Apple, aspberry, Strawberry, Raisin, Lemon, Raisin) ☛ Serving size= 1 oz, 28.4 g; GI= 63 (Medium); GL= 8.2 (Low); Net carb= 13 g

Doughnut, Yeast-Leavened With Creme Filling ☛ Serving size= 1 oz, 28.4 g; GI= 55 (Medium); GL= 4.6 (Low); Net carb= 8.3 g

Doughnut, Yeast-Leavened With Jelly Filling ☛ Serving size= 1 oz, 28.4 g; GI= 55 (Medium); GL= 5.9 (Low); Net carb= 10.8 g

Dumpling Plain ☛ Serving size= 1 small, 18 g; GI= 63 (Medium); GL= 2.2 (Low); Net carb= 3.5 g

English Muffins ☛ Serving size= 1 oz, 28.4 g; GI= 70 (High); GL= 8 (Low); Net carb= 11.4 g

English Muffins, Mixed-Grain ☛ Serving size= 1 oz, 28.4 g; GI= 71 (High); GL= 8.8 (Low); Net carb= 12.4 g

English Muffins, Plain (Includes Sourdough) ☛ Serving size= 1 oz, 28.4 g; GI= 73 (High); GL= 9 (Low); Net carb= 12.3 g

English Muffins, Whole-Wheat ☛ Serving size= 1 oz, 28.4 g; GI= 70 (High); GL= 6.7 (Low); Net carb= 9.6 g

French Toast, Frozen, Ready-To-Heat ☛ Serving size= 1 oz, 28.4 g; GI= 79 (High); GL= 7 (Low); Net carb= 8.8 g

Fritter Apple ☛ Serving size= 1 fritter (2-1/2 inch long x 1-5/8 inch wide), 17 g; GI= 61 (Medium); GL= 3.5 (Low); Net carb= 5.7 g

Fritter Banana ☛ Serving size= 1 fritter (2 inch long), 34 g; GI= 63 (Medium); GL= 6.9 (Low); Net carb= 11 g

Fritter Berry ☛ Serving size= 1 fritter (1-1/4 inch dia), 24 g; GI= 61 (Medium); GL= 4.3 (Low); Net carb= 7.1 g

Muffin, Cheese ☛ Serving size= 1 muffin, 58 g; GI= 55 (Medium); GL= 9.4 (Low); Net carb= 17 g

Muffin, Whole Grain ☛ Serving size= 1 miniature, 25 g; GI= 53 (Low); GL= 5.8 (Low); Net carb= 11 g

Muffin, Whole Wheat ☛ Serving size= 1 miniature, 25 g; GI= 51 (Low); GL= 5.2 (Low); Net carb= 10.2 g

Pancake, Blueberry Made From Recipe ☛ Serving size= 1 oz, 28.4 g; GI= 67 (Medium); GL= 5.5 (Low); Net carb= 8.2 g

Pancake, Buttermilk Made From Recipe ☛ Serving size= 1 oz, 28.4 g; GI= 67 (Medium); GL= 5.5 (Low); Net carb= 8.2 g

Pancake, Plain Frozen, Ready-To-Heat (Includes Buttermilk) ☛ Serving size= 1 oz, 28.4 g; GI= 72 (High); GL= 7.5 (Low); Net carb= 10.4 g

Pancake, Plain Made From Recipe ☛ Serving size= 1 oz, 28.4 g; GI= 67 (Medium); GL= 5.4 (Low); Net carb= 8 g

Pie, Apple Made From Recipe ☛ Serving size= 1 oz, 28.4 g; GI= 59 (Medium); GL= 6.2 (Low); Net carb= 10.5 g

Pie, Blueberry Made From Recipe ☛ Serving size= 1 oz, 28.4 g; GI= 59 (Medium); GL= 5.6 (Low); Net carb= 9.5 g

Pie, Coconut Cream ☛ Serving size= 1 oz, 28.4 g; GI= 59 (Medium); GL= 4.7 (Low); Net carb= 8 g

Pie, Egg Custard ☛ Serving size= 1 oz, 28.4 g; GI= 59 (Medium); GL= 3.2 (Low); Net carb= 5.5 g

Pie, Lemon Meringue ☛ Serving size= 1 oz, 28.4 g; GI= 59 (Medium); GL= 7.7 (Low); Net carb= 13.1 g

Pie, Pecan Made From Recipe ☛ Serving size= 1 oz, 28.4 g; GI= 59 (Medium); GL= 8.7 (Low); Net carb= 14.8 g

Roll, Dinner Wheat ☛ Serving size= 1 roll (1 oz), 28 g; GI= 77 (High); GL= 9.1 (Low); Net carb= 11.8 g

Roll, Dinner Whole-Wheat ☛ Serving size= 1 roll (1 oz), 28 g; GI= 77 (High); GL= 9.4 (Low); Net carb= 12.2 g

Waffle, Plain Frozen, Ready-To-Heat ☛ Serving size= 1 oz, 28.4 g; GI= 75 (High); GL= 8.7 (Low); Net carb= 11.6 g

Waffle, Plain Made From Recipe ☛ Serving size= 1 oz, 28.4 g; GI= 69 (Medium); GL= 6.4 (Low); Net carb= 9.3 g

BEEF, LAMP, VEAL, PORK & POULTRY

❄

Beef or Veal—Heart: Braised, Broiled, Baked, Stewed or Fried ☛ Serving size= 3 oz, 85 g; GI= 0 (Low); GL= 0 (Low); Net carb= 0 g

Beef or Veal—Bottom Round: Braised, Broiled, Baked, Stewed or Fried ☛ Serving size= 3 oz, 85 g; GI= 0 (Low); GL= 0 (Low); Net carb= 0 g

Beef or Veal—Brain: Braised, Broiled, Baked, Stewed or Fried ☛ Serving size= 3 oz, 85 g; GI= 0 (Low); GL= 0 (Low); Net carb= 0 g

Beef or Veal—Brisket: Braised, Broiled, Baked, Stewed or Fried ☛ Serving size= 3 oz, 85 g; GI= 0 (Low); GL= 0 (Low); Net carb= 0 g

Beef or Veal—Chuck Steak Varieties Chart ☛ Serving size= 3 oz, 85 g; GI= 0 (Low); GL= 0 (Low); Net carb= 0 g

Beef or Veal—Chuck Steak Varieties Chart: Braised, Broiled, Baked, Stewed or Fried ☛ Serving size= 3 oz, 85 g; GI= 0 (Low); GL= 0 (Low); Net carb= 0 g

Beef or Veal—Cuts of Steak: Braised, Broiled, Baked, Stewed or Fried ☛ Serving size= 3 oz, 85 g; GI= 0 (Low); GL= 0 (Low); Net carb= 0 g

Beef or Veal—Doner Kebab ☛ Serving size= 3 oz, 85 g; GI= 85 (High); GL= 6.4 (Low); Net carb= 7.5 g

Beef—frankfurter ☛ Serving size= 1 frankfurter, 45 g; GI= 28 (Low); GL= 0.5 (Low); Net carb= 1.8 g

Beef or Veal—Kidney: Braised, Broiled, Baked, Stewed or Fried ☛ Serving size= 3 oz, 85 g; GI= 0 (Low); GL= 0 (Low); Net carb= 0 g

Beef or Veal—Liver: Braised, Broiled, Baked, Stewed or Fried ☛ Serving size= 3 oz, 85 g; GI= 50 (Low); GL= 2.1 (Low); Net carb= 4.1 g

Beef—Tenderloin: Braised, Broiled, Baked, Stewed or Fried ☛ Serving size= 3 oz, 85 g; GI= 0 (Low); GL= 0 (Low); Net carb= 0 g

Beef or Veal—Tripe: Braised, Broiled, Baked, Stewed or Fried ☛ Serving size= 3 oz, 85 g; GI= 0 (Low); GL= 0 (Low); Net carb= 0 g

Chicken or Turkey—Backs and Necks: Braised, Broiled, Baked, Stewed or Fried ☛ Serving size= 3 oz, 85 g; GI= 0 (Low); GL= 0 (Low); Net carb= 0 g

Chicken or Turkey—Breast Fillet Tenderloin: Braised, Broiled, Baked, Stewed or Fried ☛ Serving size= 3 oz, 85 g; GI= 0 (Low); GL= 0 (Low); Net carb= 0 g

Chicken or Turkey—Drumstick: Braised, Broiled, Baked, Stewed or Fried ☛ Serving size= 3 oz, 85 g; GI= 0 (Low); GL= 0 (Low); Net carb= 0 g

Chicken or Turkey—Leg: Braised, Broiled, Baked, Stewed or Fried ☛ Serving size= 3 oz, 85 g; GI= 0 (Low); GL= 0 (Low); Net carb= 0 g

Chicken or Turkey—Tender: Braised, Broiled, Baked, Stewed or Fried ☛ Serving size= 3 oz, 85 g; GI= 0 (Low); GL= 0 (Low); Net carb= 0 g

Chicken or Turkey—Wing: Braised, Broiled, Baked, Stewed or Fried ☛ Serving size= 3 oz, 85 g; GI= 0 (Low); GL= 0 (Low); Net carb= 0 g

Eggs—Free-Range ☛ Serving size= 1 egg, 50 g; GI= (Low); GL= 0 (Low); Net carb= 0 g

Eggs—Free-Run ☛ Serving size= 1 egg, 50 g; GI= (Low); GL= 0 (Low); Net carb= 0 g

Eggs—Organic ☛ Serving size= 1 egg, 50 g; GI= (Low); GL= 0 (Low); Net carb= 0 g

Lamb—Breast: Braised, Broiled, Baked, Stewed or Fried ☛ Serving size= 3 oz, 85 g; GI= 0 (Low); GL= 0 (Low); Net carb= 0 g

Lamb—Cutlets: Braised, Broiled, Baked, Stewed or Fried ☛ Serving size= 3 oz, 85 g; GI= 0 (Low); GL= 0 (Low); Net carb= 0 g

Lamb—Leg: Braised, Broiled, Baked, Stewed or Fried ☛ Serving size= 3 oz, 85 g; GI= 0 (Low); GL= 0 (Low); Net carb= 0 g

Lamb—Loin: Braised, Broiled, Baked, Stewed or Fried ☛ Serving size= 3 oz, 85 g; GI= 0 (Low); GL= 0 (Low); Net carb= 0 g

Lamb—Shoulder: Braised, Broiled, Baked, Stewed or Fried ☛ Serving size= 3 oz, 85 g; GI= 0 (Low); GL= 0 (Low); Net carb= 0 g

Pork—back ribs: Braised, Broiled, Baked, Stewed or Fried ☛ Serving size= 3 oz, 85 g; GI= 0 (Low); GL= 0 (Low); Net carb= 0 g

Pork—Belly: Braised, Broiled, Baked, Stewed or Fried ☛ Serving size= 3 oz, 85 g; GI= 0 (Low); GL= 0 (Low); Net carb= 0 g

Pork—Cutlets: Braised, Broiled, Baked, Stewed or Fried ☛ Serving size= 3 oz, 85 g; GI= 0 (Low); GL= 0 (Low); Net carb= 0 g

Pork—Sausages: Braised, Broiled, Baked, Stewed or Fried ☛ Serving size= 3 oz, 85 g; GI= 0 (Low); GL= 0 (Low); Net carb= 0 g

BEVERAGES

❄

— **People with diabetes must avoid heavy drinking**

Acai Berry Drink ☛ Serving size= 4 fl oz, 133 g; GI= 27 (Low); GL= 4.2 (Low); Net carb= 15.5 g

100, 94, 90, 86 Proof Liquor ☛ Serving size= 1 fl oz, 27.8 g; GI= 0 (Low); GL= 0 (Low); Net carb= 0 g

Beer ☛ Serving size= 8 fl oz, 266 g; GI= 100 (High); GL= 9.4 (Low); Net carb= 9.4 g

Creme De Menthe 72 Proof ☛ Serving size= 1 fl oz, 33.6 g; GI= 63 (Medium); GL= 8.8 (Low); Net carb= 14 g

Gin, Rum, Whisky, Vodka ☛ Serving size= 1 fl oz, 27.8 g; GI= 0 (Low); GL= 0 (Low); Net carb= 0 g

Liqueur Coffee 63 Proof ☛ Serving size= 1 fl oz, 34.8 g; GI= 63 (Medium); GL= 7.1 (Low); Net carb= 11.2 g

Muscat Wine ☛ Serving size= 4 fl oz, 133 g; GI= 7 (Low); GL= 0.5 (Low); Net carb= 7 g

Red Wine ☛ Serving size= 4 fl oz, 133 g; GI= 7 (Low); GL= 0.2 (Low); Net carb= 3.5 g

Rose Wine ☛ Serving size= 4 fl oz, 133 g; GI= 7 (Low); GL= 0.4 (Low); Net carb= 5.1 g

Sauvignon Blanc ☛ Serving size= 4 fl oz, 133 g; GI= 7 (Low); GL= 0.2 (Low); Net carb= 2.7 g

Semillon ☛ Serving size= 4 fl oz, 133 g; GI= 7 (Low); GL= 0.3 (Low); Net carb= 4.1 g

Whiskey Sour ☛ Serving size= 1 fl oz, 30.4 g; GI= 73 (High); GL= 2.9 (Low); Net carb= 4 g

White Wine ☛ Serving size= 1 fl oz, 29.4 g; GI= 7 (Low); GL= 0.1 (Low); Net carb= 0.8 g

Aloe Vera Juice Drink ☛ Serving size= 8 fl oz, 266 g; GI= 66 (Medium); GL= 6.6 (Low); Net carb= 10 g

Apple Cider ☛ Serving size= 12 fl oz, 355 g; GI= 40 (Low); GL= 8.4 (Low); Net carb= 21 g

Cola Or Pepper-Type, Low Calorie ☛ Serving size= 8 fl oz, 266 g; GI= 54 (Low); GL= 0.4 (Low); Net carb= 0.8 g

Limeade High Caffeine ☛ Serving size= 8 fl oz, 266 g; GI= 68 (Medium); GL= 7.4 (Low); Net carb= 10.9 g

Carbonated Drink, Other Than Cola Or Pepper, Low Calorie With Aspartame ☛ Serving size= 8 fl oz, 266 g; GI= 54 (Low); GL= 0 (Low); Net carb= 0 g

Chicory Beverage ☛ Serving size= 8 fl oz, 266 g; GI= 9 (Low); GL= 0.3 (Low); Net carb= 3.8 g

Chocolate Almond Milk ☛ Serving size= 4 fl oz, 133 g; GI= 35 (Low); GL= 4.2 (Low); Net carb= 11.9 g

Citrus Green Tea ☛ Serving size= 8 fl oz, 266 g; GI= 0 (Low); GL= 0

(Low); Net carb= 0.8 g

Coconut Water—Ready-To-Drink—Unsweetened ☛ Serving size= 8 fl oz, 266 g; GI= 41 (Low); GL= 4.6 (Low); Net carb= 11.3 g

Coffee ☛ Serving size= 1 fl oz, 29.6 g; GI= 0 (Low); GL= 0 (Low); Net carb= 0 g

Coffee Instant, Chicory ☛ Serving size= 1 fl oz, 29.9 g; GI= 7 (Low); GL= 0 (Low); Net carb= 0.2 g

Coffee Instant, Mocha Sweetened ☛ Serving size= 1 serving 2 tbsp, 13 g; GI= 89 (High); GL= 8.4 (Low); Net carb= 9.4 g

Coffee, Bottled or canned, Light ☛ Serving size= 1 fl oz, 30 g; GI= 21 (Low); GL= 0.4 (Low); Net carb= 1.8 g

Coffee, Brewed ☛ Serving size= 1 fl oz, 29.6 g; GI= 0 (Low); GL= 0 (Low); Net carb= 0.5 g

Coffee, Cafe Con Leche ☛ Serving size= 1 fl oz, 31 g; GI= 5 (Low); GL= 0.1 (Low); Net carb= 1.7 g

Coffee, Cafe Mocha ☛ Serving size= 1 fl oz, 31 g; GI= 21 (Low); GL= 0.7 (Low); Net carb= 3.1 g

Coffee, Cappuccino ☛ Serving size= 1 fl oz, 30 g; GI= 33 (Low); GL= 0.3 (Low); Net carb= 0.8 g

Coffee, Cuban ☛ Serving size= 1 fl oz, 31 g; GI= 41 (Low); GL= 1 (Low); Net carb= 2.4 g

Coffee, Latte ☛ Serving size= 1 fl oz, 30 g; GI= 21 (Low); GL= 0.3 (Low); Net carb= 1.3 g

Coffee, Macchiato ☛ Serving size= 1 fl oz, 30 g; GI= 21 (Low); GL= 0.2 (Low); Net carb= 0.8 g

Coffee, Turkish ☛ Serving size= 1 fl oz, 31 g; GI= 51 (Low); GL= 1 (Low); Net carb= 2 g

Diet Cola ☛ Serving size= 8 fl oz, 266 g; GI= 41 (Low); GL= 5.6

(Low); Net carb= 13.7 g

Diet Pepper Cola ➡ Serving size= 8 fl oz, 266 g; GI= 11 (Low); GL= 0 (Low); Net carb= 0.3 g

Energy Drink, Low Carb Monster ➡ Serving size= 8 fl oz, 266 g; GI= 15 (Low); GL= 0.6 (Low); Net carb= 3.7 g

Energy Drink, Red Bull Sugar Free ➡ Serving size= 8 fl oz, 266 g; GI= 0 (Low); GL= 0 (Low); Net carb= 1.9 g

Energy Drink, Rockstar Sugar Free ➡ Serving size= 8 fl oz, 266 g; GI= 0 (Low); GL= 0 (Low); Net carb= 1.9 g

Energy Drink, Sugar Free ➡ Serving size= 8 fl oz, 266 g; GI= 0 (Low); GL= 0 (Low); Net carb= 1.1 g

Fruit Flavored Smoothie Drink Frozen Light No Dairy ➡ Serving size= 8 fl oz, 266 g; GI= 68 (Medium); GL= 5.8 (Low); Net carb= 8.5 g

Lemonade—Powder Made With Water ➡ Serving size= 8 fl oz, 266 g; GI= 68 (Medium); GL= 6.5 (Low); Net carb= 9.5 g

Rich Chocolate Powder ➡ Serving size= 2 tbsp, 11 g; GI= 89 (High); GL= 9.1 (Low); Net carb= 10.2 g

Soy Protein Powder ➡ Serving size= 1 scoop, 44 g; GI= 47 (Low); GL= 9.1 (Low); Net carb= 19.3 g

Tap Water ➡ Serving size= 8 fl oz, 266 g; GI= 0 (Low); GL= 0 (Low); Net carb= 0 g

Tea Green or Black, Brewed, or Ready-to-Drink ➡ Serving size= 1 cup, 245 g; GI= 0 (Low); GL= 0 (Low); Net carb= 0 g

Tea Herb, Brewed ➡ Serving size= 1 fl oz, 29.6 g; GI= 0 (Low); GL= 0 (Low); Net carb= 0.1 g

Whey Protein Powder ➡ Serving size= 2 scoop, 39 g; GI= 47 (Low); GL= 3.3 (Low); Net carb= 7 g

CONDIMENTS, OILS & SAUCES

Alfredo Sauce ▸ Serving size= ¼ cup, 62 g; GI= 27 (Low); GL= 0.4 (Low); Net carb= 1.6 g

Beef Tallow ▸ Serving size= 1 tbsp, 15 g; GI= 0 (Low); GL= 0 (Low); Net carb= 0 g

Clarified Butter ▸ Serving size= 1 tbsp, 15 g; GI= 0 (Low); GL= 0 (Low); Net carb= 0 g

Cocktail sauce ▸ Serving size= ¼ cup, 62 g; GI= 38 (Low); GL= 6.8 (Low); Net carb= 18 g

Dressing—Blue or roquefort ▸ Serving size= 2 tbsp, 30 g; GI= 50 (Low); GL= 4.1 (Low); Net carb= 8.1 g

Dressing—Blue or roquefort, reduced calorie ▸ Serving size= 2 tbsp, 30 g; GI= 5 (Low); GL= 0 (Low); Net carb= 0.9 g

Dressing—Caesar ▸ Serving size= ¼ cup, 62 g; GI= 50 (Low); GL= 0.8 (Low); Net carb= 1.6 g

Dressing—Coleslaw ▸ Serving size= ¼ cup, 62 g; GI= 50 (Low); GL= 1.2 (Low); Net carb= 2.3 g

Dressing—Coleslaw, reduced calorie ☛ Serving size= ¼ cup, 62 g; GI= 5 (Low); GL= 0 (Low); Net carb= 0 g

Dressing—Cream cheese ☛ Serving size= 2 tbsp, 30 g; GI= 50 (Low); GL= 0.5 (Low); Net carb= 1 g

Dressing—Feta Cheese ☛ Serving size= ¼ cup, 62 g; GI= 50 (Low); GL= 0.7 (Low); Net carb= 1.4 g

Dressing—French ☛ Serving size= 2 tbsp, 30 g; GI= 50 (Low); GL= 4.5 (Low); Net carb= 9 g

Dressing—French, reduced calorie, fat free ☛ Serving size= 2 tbsp, 30 g; GI= 50 (Low); GL= 1.9 (Low); Net carb= 3.8 g

Dressing—Honey mustard ☛ Serving size= 2 tbsp, 30 g; GI= 50 (Low); GL= 4.2 (Low); Net carb= 8.4 g

Dressing—Italian ☛ Serving size= 2 tbsp, 30 g; GI= 50 (Low); GL= 1.1 (Low); Net carb= 2.2 g

Dressing—Korean ☛ Serving size= ¼ cup, 62 g; GI= 50 (Low); GL= 1.9 (Low); Net carb= 3.7 g

Dressing—Mayonnaise-type salad ☛ Serving size= 2 tbsp, 30 g; GI= 50 (Low); GL= 3 (Low); Net carb= 6 g

Dressing—Mayonnaise-type salad, diet ☛ Serving size= 2 tbsp, 30 g; GI= 50 (Low); GL= 1.1 (Low); Net carb= 2.2 g

Dressing—Peppercorn ☛ Serving size= 2 tbsp, 30 g; GI= 50 (Low); GL= 1 (Low); Net carb= 2 g

Dressing—Poppy seed ☛ Serving size= 2 tbsp, 30 g; GI= 50 (Low); GL= 3.1 (Low); Net carb= 6.2 g

Dressing—Rice ☛ Serving size= 2 tbsp, 30 g; GI= 64 (Low); GL= 3.4 (Low); Net carb= 5.3 g

Dressing—Russian ☛ Serving size= 2 tbsp, 30 g; GI= 50 (Low); GL= 4.8 (Low); Net carb= 9.6 g

Dressing—Salad, common ☛ Serving size= 2 tbsp, 30 g; GI= 50 (Low); GL= 1.4 (Low); Net carb= 2.8 g

Dressing—Thousand Island Regular ☛ Serving size= 2 tbsp, 30 g; GI= 50 (Low); GL= 1.5 (Low); Net carb= 2.9 g

Dressing—Vinegar based ☛ Serving size= ¼ cup, 62 g; GI= 50 (Low); GL= 0.8 (Low); Net carb= 1.6 g

Dressing—Yogurt ☛ Serving size= ¼ cup, 62 g; GI= 50 (Low); GL= 1.9 (Low); Net carb= 3.8 g

Mayonnaise (mean value) ☛ Serving size= 2 tbsp, 30 g; GI= 50 (Low); GL= 1.2 (Low); Net carb= 2.4 g

Mayonnaise—made with tofu ☛ Serving size= 2 tbsp, 30 g; GI= 50 (Low); GL= 0.3 (Low); Net carb= 0.6 g

Mustard greens (mean value) ☛ Serving size= 2 tbsp, 30 g; GI= 32 (Low); GL= 0.2 (Low); Net carb= 0.5 g

Oil—Avocado, Canola, Coconut, Corn, Flaxseed, Grapeseed, Hazelnut, Or Hemp seed ☛ Serving size= 2 tbsp, 30 g; GI= 0 (Low); GL= 0 (Low); Net carb= 0 g

Oil—Extra-virgin olive, Olive ☛ Serving size= 2 tbsp, 30 g; GI= 0 (Low); GL= 0 (Low); Net carb= 0 g

Oil—Macadamia Nut, Palm, Peanut, Sesame, Sunflower Or Walnut ☛ Serving size= 2 tbsp, 30 g; GI= 0 (Low); GL= 0 (Low); Net carb= 0 g

Vinegar, sugar, and water dressing ☛ Serving size= 2 tbsp, 30 g; GI= 0 (Low); GL= 0 (Low); Net carb= 0 g

DAIRY AND SOY ALTERNATIVES

Butter, Or Butter-vegetable oil blend ☛ Serving size: 1 tsp (4.7 g); GI= 50 (Low); GL= 0.3 (Low); Net carb= 0.6 g

Buttermilk, fluid ☛ Serving size: 1 cup (245 g); GI= 29.5 (Low); GL= 3.6 (Low); Net carb= 12.2 g

Cheese Soy ☛ Serving size: 1 oz (28.35 g); GI= 40 (Low); GL= 2.7 (Low); Net carb= 6.8 g

Cheese, Blue, Roquefort, Edam, Feta, Fontina, Goat, Gouda, Gruyere, Monterey, American style (average value) ☛ Serving size: 1 oz (28.35 g); GI= 27 (Low); GL= 0.2 (Low); Net carb= 0.7 g

Cheese, camembert, Cheddar, Colby, Limburger, Manchego ☛ Serving size: 1 oz (28.35 g); GI= 25 (Low); GL= 0.2 (Low); Net carb= 0.8 g

Cheese, cottage, Swiss (average value) ☛ Serving size: 1 oz (28.35 g); GI= 29.5 (Low); GL= 0.3 (Low); Net carb= 1 g

Cheese, cream ☛ Serving size: 1 oz (28.35 g); GI= 27 (Low); GL= 2.3 (Low); Net carb= 8.5 g

Cheese, Monterey, Mozzarella, Muenster, Parmesan, Provolone, Pecorino Romano, Ricotta ☛ Serving size: 1 oz (28.35 g); GI= 27 (Low); GL= 0.2 (Low); Net carb= 0.7 g

Cream, light, fluid, or whipped ☛ Serving size: 1 oz (28.35 g); GI= 27 (Low); GL= 2.3 (Low); Net carb= 8.5 g

Custard homemade, or Puerto Rican style (average value) ☛ Serving size: ½ cup (116 g); GI= 29 (Low); GL= 6.7 (Low); Net carb= 23.1 g

Ghee ☛ Serving size: 1 tsp (4.7 g); GI= 0.0 (Low); GL= 0 (Low); Net carb= 0 g

Ice cream—average value ☛ Serving size: 1 scoop (72 g); GI= 64.5 (Medium); GL= 7.9 (Low); Net carb= 12.2 g

Kefir ☛ Serving size: 1 cup (245 g); GI= 32 (Low); GL= 0.7 (Low); Net carb= 2.2 g

Margarine ☛ Serving size: 1 tsp (4.7 g); GI= 50 (Low); GL= 0 (Low); Net carb= 0 g

Milk beverage, With flavors, low-calorie sweetener (average value) ☛ Serving size: 1 cup (245 g); GI= 24 (Low); GL= 2.6 (Low); Net carb= 10.8 g

Milk lactose free ☛ Serving size: 1 cup (245 g); GI= 40 (Low); GL= 6 (Low); Net carb= 15 g

Milk made from soy protein ☛ Serving size: 1 cup (245 g); GI= 50 (Low); GL= 7.4 (Low); Net carb= 14.8 g

Milk, almond ☛ Serving size: 1 cup (245 g); GI= 25 (Low); GL= 2 (Low); Net carb= 8 g

Milk, chocolate, regular (average value) ☛ Serving size: 1 cup (245 g); GI= 37 (Low); GL= 9.1 (Low); Net carb= 24.6 g

Milk, coconut ☛ Serving size: 1 cup (245 g); GI= 41 (Low); GL= 6 (Low); Net carb= 14.6 g

Milk, Cow's, whole, skim or reduced fat ☛ Serving size: 1 cup (245 g); GI= 40 (Low); GL= 4.8 (Low); Net carb= 12 g

Milk, dry, reconstituted (average value) ☛ Serving size: 1 cup (245 g); GI= 32 (Low); GL= 3.8 (Low); Net carb= 11.9 g

Milk, Goat's, whole ☛ Serving size: 1 cup (245 g); GI= 40 (Low); GL= 4.4 (Low); Net carb= 11 g

Milk, hemp ☛ Serving size: 1 cup (245 g); GI= 0.0 (Low); GL= 0 (Low); Net carb= 0 g

Milk, malted (average value) ☛ Serving size: 1 cup (245 g); GI= 45 (Low); GL= 5.4 (Low); Net carb= 12 g

Milk, soy based, dry, reconstituted or ready-to-drink (average) ☛ Serving size: 1 cup (245 g); GI= 40 (Low); GL= 5.9 (Low); Net carb= 14.8 g

Pudding, pumpkin ☛ Serving size: 4 oz (120 g); GI= 47 (Low); GL= 9.4 (Low); Net carb= 20 g

Traditional Greek yoghurt ☛ Serving size: 1 cup (245 g); GI= 0.0 (Low); GL= 0 (Low); Net carb= 0 g

Yoghurt, Goat's milk ☛ Serving size: 8 oz (225 g); GI= 25 (Low); GL= 2.75 (Low); Net carb= 11 g

Yoghurt, lactose free ☛ Serving size: 1 cup (245 g); GI= 50 (Low); GL= 4.9 (Low); Net carb= 9.8 g

Yoghurt, natural low-fat, regular (average) ☛ Serving size: 1 cup (245 g); GI= 50 (Low); GL= 4.9 (Low); Net carb= 9.8 g

Yogurt, fruit variety ☛ Serving size: 1 cup (245 g); GI= 31 (Low); GL= 3 (Low); Net carb= 9.7 g

Yogurt, plain ☛ Serving size: 1 cup (245 g); GI= 36 (Low); GL= 3.5 (Low); Net carb= 9.7 g

LEGUMS AND BEANS

Adzuki Beans, Cooked ➤ Serving size= ½ cup, 150 g; GI= 33 (Low); GL= 8.6 (Low); Net carb= 26.2 g

Baked Beans, Canned, Cooked (average) ➤ Serving size= ½ cup, 150 g; GI= 40 (Low); GL= 9.7 (Low); Net carb= 24.2 g

Bayo Beans, Dry Cooked ➤ Serving size= ½ cup, 150 g; GI= 30 (Low); GL= 6.7 (Low); Net carb= 22.3 g

Black Beans, Cooked ➤ Serving size= ½ cup, 150 g; GI= 30 (Low); GL= 6.8 (Low); Net carb= 22.5 g

Black Turtle Beans, Canned, Drained ➤ Serving size= ½ cup, 150 g; GI= 41 (Low); GL= 5.9 (Low); Net carb= 14.5 g

Black Turtle Beans, Cooked ➤ Serving size= ½ cup, 150 g; GI= 41 (Low); GL= 9.9 (Low); Net carb= 24.1 g

Broad Beans (Fava) ➤ Serving size= ½ cup, 150 g; GI= 40 (Low); GL= 8.6 (Low); Net carb= 21.4 g

Broad beans (Fava), Canned, Drained ➤ Serving size= ½ cup, 150 g; GI= 40 (Low); GL= 5.2 (Low); Net carb= 13.1 g

California Red Kidney Beans ☞ Serving size= ½ cup, 150 g; GI= 33 (Low); GL= 6.5 (Low); Net carb= 19.7 g

Chickpeas (Garbanzo), Dry Cooked ☞ Serving size= ½ cup, 150 g; GI= 36 (Low); GL= 9.9 (Low); Net carb= 27.4 g

Chickpeas (Garbanzo), Canned Drained Rinsed ☞ Serving size= ½ cup, 150 g; GI= 36 (Low); GL= 8.9 (Low); Net carb= 24.9 g

Cowpeas, Dry Cooked ☞ Serving size= ½ cup, 150 g; GI= 50 (Low); GL= 9.8 (Low); Net carb= 19.7 g

Cowpeas, Canned Plain ☞ Serving size= ½ cup, 150 g; GI= 50 (Low); GL= 7.7 (Low); Net carb= 15.5 g

Edamame ☞ Serving size= ½ cup, 150 g; GI= 20 (Low); GL= 1.1 (Low); Net carb= 5.6 g

Extra Firm Tofu ☞ Serving size= ½ cup, 150 g; GI= 15 (Low); GL= 0.2 (Low); Net carb= 1.2 g

French Beans, Cooked ☞ Serving size= ½ cup, 150 g; GI= 21 (Low); GL= 4.6 (Low); Net carb= 21.9 g

Green Soybeans ☞ Serving size= ½ cup, 150 g; GI= 18 (Low); GL= 1.8 (Low); Net carb= 10.3 g

Hummus (Commercial) ☞ Serving size= 10 tbsp, 150 g; GI= 15 (Low); GL= 2 (Low); Net carb= 14 g

Hummus (Homemade) ☞ Serving size= 10 tbsp, 150 g; GI= 15 (Low); GL= 4 (Low); Net carb= 24 g

Kidney Beans, Cooked (average) ☞ Serving size= ½ cup, 150 g; GI= 33 (Low); GL= 7.6 (Low); Net carb= 23.1 g

Lentils, Dry Cooked ☞ Serving size= ½ cup, 150 g; GI= 21 (Low); GL= 3.8 (Low); Net carb= 18.2 g

Lima Beans, Dry Cooked ☞ Serving size= ½ cup, 150 g; GI= 46 (Low); GL= 9.5 (Low); Net carb= 20.7 g

Miso ☛ Serving size= 1 tbsp, 17 g; GI= 63 (Medium); GL= 2.1 (Low); Net carb= 3.4 g

Mung Beans, Dry Cooked ☛ Serving size= ½ cup, 150 g; GI= 42 (Low); GL= 7.2 (Low); Net carb= 17.2 g

Natto ☛ Serving size= ½ cup, 150 g; GI= 54 (Low); GL= 5.9 (Low); Net carb= 10.9 g

Navy Beans, Cooked ☛ Serving size= ½ cup, 150 g; GI= 39 (Low); GL= 9.1 (Low); Net carb= 23.3 g

Okara ☛ Serving size= 1 cup, 122 g; GI= 53 (Low); GL= 7.9 (Low); Net carb= 14.9 g

Peanut Butter, Chunk Style Or Smooth (average) ☛ Serving size= 2 tbsp, 32 g; GI= 14 (Low); GL= 0.8 (Low); Net carb= 5.8 g

Peanuts, Spanish Raw ☛ Serving size= 1 cup, 146 g; GI= 13 (Low); GL= 1.2 (Low); Net carb= 9.2 g

Peanuts, Valencia Raw ☛ Serving size= 1 cup, 146 g; GI= 13 (Low); GL= 2.3 (Low); Net carb= 17.8 g

Peas, Dry Cooked ☛ Serving size= ½ cup, 150 g; GI= 22 (Low); GL= 3.5 (Low); Net carb= 16 g

Split Peas, Cooked ☛ Serving size= ½ cup, 150 g; GI= 51 (Low); GL= 9.3 (Low); Net carb= 18.3 g

Split Peas, Green Or Yellow, Dry Cooked ☛ Serving size= ½ cup, 150 g; GI= 33 (Low); GL= 6.3 (Low); Net carb= 19 g

Pigeon Peas—Mature Seeds Cooked ☛ Serving size= ½ cup, 150 g; GI= 31 (Low); GL= 7.7 (Low); Net carb= 24.8 g

Pinto Beans, Canned Drained, Cooked ☛ Serving size= ½ cup, 150 g; GI= 39 (Low); GL= 8.6 (Low); Net carb= 22.1 g

Red Kidney Beans, Canned Drained, Cooked ☛ Serving size= ½ cup, 150 g; GI= 35 (Low); GL= 8.8 (Low); Net carb= 25.1 g

Red Kidney Beans, Dry Cooked ☞ Serving size= ½ cup, 150 g; GI= 35 (Low); GL= 8 (Low); Net carb= 22.9 g

Small White Beans, Cooked ☞ Serving size= ½ cup, 150 g; GI= 36 (Low); GL= 8.3 (Low); Net carb= 23.1 g

Soft Tofu ☞ Serving size= 1 piece (2 1/2 inch * 2 ¾ inch * 1 inch), 120 g; GI= 15 (Low); GL= 0.2 (Low); Net carb= 1.2 g

Soy Flour (average value) ☞ Serving size= 1 cup, stirred, 84 g; GI= 25 (Low); GL= 4.7 (Low); Net carb= 18.7 g

Soy Protein, Isolate ☞ Serving size= 1 oz, 28.4 g; GI= 47 (Low); GL= 0.2 (Low); Net carb= 0.5 g

Soy Protein, Powder ☞ Serving size= 1 oz, 28.4 g; GI= 47 (Low); GL= 0.8 (Low); Net carb= 1.6 g

Soybeans, Dry Cooked ☞ Serving size= 1 cup, 180 g; GI= 31 (Low); GL= 1.3 (Low); Net carb= 4.2 g

Tamari ☞ Serving size= 1 tbsp, 18 g; GI= 20 (Low); GL= 0.2 (Low); Net carb= 0.9 g

Tempeh ☞ Serving size= 1 cup, 166 g; GI= 15 (Low); GL= 1.9 (Low); Net carb= 12.7 g

Tofu Silken Extra Firm ☞ Serving size= 1 slice, 84 g; GI= 15 (Low); GL= 0.2 (Low); Net carb= 1.6 g

Tofu Silken Firm ☞ Serving size= 1 slice, 84 g; GI= 15 (Low); GL= 0.3 (Low); Net carb= 1.9 g

White Beans—Mature Seeds Canned ☞ Serving size= ½ cup, 150 g; GI= 36 (Low); GL= 8.9 (Low); Net carb= 24.6 g

Yellow Beans—Mature Seeds Cooked ☞ Serving size= ½ cup, 150 g; GI= 36 (Low); GL= 8 (Low); Net carb= 22.3 g

FISH & FISH PRODUCTS

Fish are part of the glycemic load eating pattern and provide high-quality proteins and good fats (Omega-3 and omega-6 fats) in addition to some key nutrients such as

• vitamin B2

• calcium and phosphorus

• iron

• iodine and choline

The glycemic load of raw fish is equal to zero.

Breading or battering fish should be avoided, especially when using simple carbohydrates such as white flour. Grilling, baking, broiling, poaching, or steaming fish is considered healthier since it does not rise the glycemic index of cooked fish.

Fish, raw ☛ Serving size= 1 fillet (150 g); GI= 0 (Low); GL= 0 (Low)

Fish, canned, oil or water ☛ Serving size= 3 Oz (85 g); GI= 0 (Low); GL= 0 (Low)

Fish, smoked or pickled ☛ Serving size= 1 fillet (150 g); GI= 0 (Low); GL= 0 (Low)

Fish, cooked, without flour ☛ Serving size= 3 Oz (85 g); GI= 0 (Low); GL= 0 (Low)

Fish, floured, breaded or battered AND baked ☛ Serving size= 3 Oz (85 g); GI= 95 (High); GL= 7.8 (Low)

Fish, floured, breaded or battered AND fried ☛ Serving size= 3 Oz (85 g); GI= 95 (High); GL= 7.8 (Low)

Fish, steamed or poached ☛ Serving size= 3 Oz (85 g); GI= 0 (Low); GL= 0 (Low)

FRUITS AND FRUITS PRODUCTS

Apple Baked, unsweetened ☞ Serving size= 1 apple with liquid, 161 (g); GI= 38 (Low); GL= 7.5 (Low); Net carbs= 19.7 g

Apple Chips ☞ Serving size= 1 cup, 28 (g); GI= 35 (Low); GL= 6.3 (Low); Net carbs= 17.9 g

Apple Pickled ☞ Serving size= 1 apple, 29 (g); GI= 38 (Low); GL= 3.4 (Low); Net carbs= 8.8 g

Apple Rings Fried ☞ Serving size= 1 ring, 19 (g); GI= 38 (Low); GL= 1.2 (Low); Net carbs= 3.2 g

Apples, Raw ☞ Serving size= 1 cup, quartered or chopped, 125 (g); GI= 38 (Low); GL= 5.4 (Low); Net carbs= 14.3 g

Applesauce, Canned, unsweetened ☞ Serving size= 1 cup, 244 (g); GI= 38 (Low); GL= 9.4 (Low); Net carbs= 24.8 g

Apricot Dried Cooked Without Sugar ☞ Serving size= 1/4 cup, 67.5 (g); GI= 41 (Low); GL= 7.8 (High); Net carbs= 19 g

Apricots ☞ Serving size= 1 cup, halves, 155 (g); GI= 31 (Low); GL= 4.4 (Low); Net carbs= 14.1 g

Asian Pears ☛ Serving size= 1 fruit, 122 (g); GI= 26 (Low); GL= 2.2 (Low); Net carbs= 8.6 g

Avocados ☛ Serving size= 1 cup, cubes, 150 (g); GI= 50 (Low); GL= 1.4 (Low); Net carbs= 2.7 g

Avocados ☛ Serving size= 1 cup, pureed, 230 (g); GI= 50 (Low); GL= 2.6 (Low); Net carbs= 5.1 g

Banana, Ripe Fried ☛ Serving size= 1 small, 73 (g); GI= 62 (Medium); GL= 9.6 (Low); Net carbs= 15.5 g

Bartlett Pears ☛ Serving size= 1 cup, sliced, 140 (g); GI= 41 (Low); GL= 6.8 (Low); Net carbs= 16.7 g

Blackberries, Raw or Frozen ☛ Serving size= 1 cup, 144 (g); GI= 25 (Low); GL= 1.6 (Low); Net carbs= 6.2 g

Blueberries, Raw or Frozen ☛ Serving size= 1 cup, 148 (g); GI= 53 (Low); GL= 9.5 (Low); Net carbs= 17.9 g

Bosc Pear, Raw or Frozen ☛ Serving size= 1 cup, sliced, 140 (g); GI= 41 (Low); GL= 7.5 (Low); Net carbs= 18.2 g

Boysenberries, Raw or Frozen ☛ Serving size= 1 cup, unthawed, 132 (g); GI= 43 (Low); GL= 3.9 (Low); Net carbs= 9.1 g

California Avocados ☛ Serving size= 1 cup, pureed, 230 (g); GI= 50 (Low); GL= 2.1 (Low); Net carbs= 4.2 g

Cantaloupe Melons ☛ Serving size= 1 cup, balls, 177 (g); GI= 61 (Medium); GL= 7.8 (Low); Net carbs= 12.9 g

Casaba Melon ☛ Serving size= 1 cup, cubes, 170 (g); GI= 62 (Medium); GL= 6 (Low); Net carbs= 9.7 g

Cherries (Sweet) ☛ Serving size= 1 cup, with pits, yields, 138 (g); GI= 22 (Low); GL= 4.2 (Low); Net carbs= 19.2 g

Clementines ☛ Serving size= 1 fruit, 74 (g); GI= 35 (Low); GL= 2.7 (Low); Net carbs= 7.6 g

Cranberries ☞ Serving size= 1 cup, chopped, 110 (g); GI= 45 (Low); GL= 4.1 (Low); Net carbs= 9.2 g

Dates, Deglet Noor ☞ Serving size= 1/5 cup, chopped, 30 (g); GI= 44 (Low); GL= 8.7 (Low); Net carbs= 19.6 g

Dates, Medjool ☞ Serving size= 1 date, pitted, 24 (g); GI= 44 (Low); GL= 7.2 (Low); Net carbs= 16.4 g

Dried Litchis ☞ Serving size= 1 fruit, 2.5 (g); GI= 60 (Medium); GL= 1 (Low); Net carbs= 1.7 g

European Black Currants ☞ Serving size= 1 cup, 112 (g); GI= 22 (Low); GL= 3.8 (Low); Net carbs= 17.2 g

Figs ☞ Serving size= 1 large (2-1/2 inch dia), 64 (g); GI= 51 (Low); GL= 5.3 (Low); Net carbs= 10.4 g

Fruit Salad, Fresh Or Raw Including Citrus Fruits No Dressing ☞ Serving size= 1 cup, 170 (g); GI= 51 (Low); GL= 9.8 (Low); Net carbs= 19.7 g

Fuji Apples ☞ Serving size= 1 cup, sliced, 109 (g); GI= 36 (Low); GL= 5.1 (Low); Net carbs= 14.3 g

Gala Apples, or Golden Delicious Apples (average) ☞ Serving size= 1 cup, sliced, 109 (g); GI= 39 (Low); GL= 4.8 (Low); Net carbs= 12.4 g

Gooseberries ☞ Serving size= 1 cup, 150 (g); GI= 21 (Low); GL= 1.9 (Low); Net carbs= 8.8 g

Granny Smith Apples ☞ Serving size= 1 cup, sliced, 109 (g); GI= 36 (Low); GL= 4.2 (Low); Net carbs= 11.8 g

Grapefruit ☞ Serving size= 1 cup sections, with juice, 230 (g); GI= 25 (Low); GL= 3.7 (Low); Net carbs= 14.7 g

Grapefruit ☞ Serving size= 1 cup sections, with juice, 230 (g); GI= 25 (Low); GL= 4 (Low); Net carbs= 16.1 g

Grapes ☛ Serving size= 1 cup, 92 (g); GI= 53 (Low); GL= 7.9 (Low); Net carbs= 15 g

Green Olives Marinated ☛ Serving size= 1 olive, 2.7 (g); GI= 17 (Low); GL= 0 (Low); Net carbs= 0 g

Groundcherries ☛ Serving size= 1 cup, 140 (g); GI= 35 (Low); GL= 5.5 (Low); Net carbs= 15.7 g

Guavas ☛ Serving size= 1 cup, 165 (g); GI= 24 (Low); GL= 3.5 (Low); Net carbs= 14.7 g

Honeydew Melon ☛ Serving size= 1 cup, diced, 170 (g); GI= 62 (Medium); GL= 8.7 (Low); Net carbs= 14.1 g

Java Plum ☛ Serving size= 1 cup, 135 (g); GI= 25 (Low); GL= 5.3 (Low); Net carbs= 21 g

Kumquats ☛ Serving size= 1 fruit without refuse, 19 (g); GI= 0 (Low); GL= 0 (Low); Net carbs= 1.8 g

Lemon Juice, Raw ☛ Serving size= 1 cup, 244 (g); GI= 51 (Low); GL= 8.2 (Low); Net carbs= 16.1 g

Lime Juice ☛ Serving size= 1 cup, 242 (g); GI= 51 (Low); GL= 9.9 (Low); Net carbs= 19.4 g

Limes ☛ Serving size= 1 fruit (2 inch dia), 67 (g); GI= 25 (Low); GL= 1.3 (Low); Net carbs= 5.2 g

Lychee, Canned in Syrup, Drained ☛ Serving size= 1 lychee with liquid, 21 (g); GI= 74 (High); GL= 3.6 (Low); Net carbs= 4.9 g

Mango Pickled ☛ Serving size= 1 slice, 28 (g); GI= 51 (Low); GL= 4.5 (Low); Net carbs= 8.9 g

Melon Balls ☛ Serving size= 1 cup, unthawed, 173 (g); GI= 62 (Medium); GL= 7.8 (Low); Net carbs= 12.5 g

Mulberries ☛ Serving size= 1 cup, 140 (g); GI= (); GL= 0 (Low); Net carbs= 11.3 g

Nance, Canned in Syrup, Drained ☛ Serving size= 3 fruit without pits, 11.1 (g); GI= 85 (High); GL= 1.5 (Low); Net carbs= 1.8 g

Navel Oranges ☛ Serving size= 1 cup sections, 165 (g); GI= 43 (Low); GL= 7.3 (Low); Net carbs= 17.1 g

Nectarines ☛ Serving size= 1 cup slices, 143 (g); GI= 35 (Low); GL= 4.4 (Low); Net carbs= 12.7 g

Olives (average value) ☛ Serving size= 1 tbsp, 8.4 (g); GI= 15 (Low); GL= 0.1 (Low); Net carbs= 0.4 g

Olives Green Stuffed ☛ Serving size= 1 cup, 147 (g); GI= 15 (Low); GL= 0.2 (Low); Net carbs= 1.4 g

Oranges ☛ Serving size= 1 cup sections, without membranes, 185 (g); GI= 42 (Low); GL= 7.1 (Low); Net carbs= 16.9 g

Oranges ☛ Serving size= 1 cup, sections, 180 (g); GI= 45 (Low); GL= 7.6 (Low); Net carbs= 16.8 g

Oranges Raw With Peel ☛ Serving size= 1 cup, 170 (g); GI= 45 (Low); GL= 8.4 (Low); Net carbs= 18.7 g

Papaya ☛ Serving size= 1 cup 1 inch pieces, 145 (g); GI= 60 (Medium); GL= 7.9 (Low); Net carbs= 13.2 g

Passion Fruit (Granadilla) ☛ Serving size= 1 cup, 236 (g); GI= 30 (Low); GL= 9.2 (Low); Net carbs= 30.6 g

Peach Pickled ☛ Serving size= 1 fruit, 88 (g); GI= 40 (Low); GL= 9.9 (Low); Net carbs= 24.8 g

Pears ☛ Serving size= 1 cup, slices, 140 (g); GI= 33 (Low); GL= 5.6 (Low); Net carbs= 17 g

Persimmons, Raw ☛ Serving size= 1 fruit without refuse, 25 (g); GI= 61 (Medium); GL= 5.1 (Low); Net carbs= 8.4 g

Plum Pickled ☛ Serving size= 1 plum, 28 (g); GI= 24 (Low); GL= 2 (Low); Net carbs= 8.3 g

Plums ☛ Serving size= 1 cup, sliced, 165 (g); GI= 24 (Low); GL= 4 (Low); Net carbs= 16.5 g

Pomegranates ☛ Serving size= 1/2 cup arils (seed/juice sacs), 87 (g); GI= 53 (Low); GL= 6.8 (Low); Net carbs= 12.8 g

Prune, Raw ☛ Serving size= 2 tbsp, 36 (g); GI= 43 (Low); GL= 9.6 (Low); Net carbs= 22.2 g

Pummelo ☛ Serving size= 1 cup, sections, 190 (g); GI= 22 (Low); GL= 3.6 (Low); Net carbs= 16.4 g

Quinces ☛ Serving size= 1 fruit without refuse, 92 (g); GI= 35 (Low); GL= 4.3 (Low); Net carbs= 12.3 g

Raspberries, Raw or frozen ☛ Serving size= 1 cup, 123 (g); GI= 78 (High); GL= 5.2 (Low); Net carbs= 6.7 g

Red And White Currants ☛ Serving size= 1 cup, 112 (g); GI= 25 (Low); GL= 2.7 (Low); Net carbs= 10.6 g

Red Delicious Apples ☛ Serving size= 1 cup, sliced, 109 (g); GI= 39 (Low); GL= 5 (Low); Net carbs= 12.8 g

Rhubarb ☛ Serving size= 1 cup, diced, 122 (g); GI= 15 (Low); GL= 0.5 (Low); Net carbs= 3.3 g

Sour Red Cherries ☛ Serving size= 1 cup, without pits, 155 (g); GI= 22 (Low); GL= 3.6 (Low); Net carbs= 16.4 g

Starfruit (Carambola) ☛ Serving size= 1 cup, cubes, 132 (g); GI= 45 (Low); GL= 2.3 (Low); Net carbs= 5.2 g

Strawberries ☛ Serving size= 1 cup, halves, 152 (g); GI= 41 (Low); GL= 3.5 (Low); Net carbs= 8.6 g

Tangerines Juices Canned ☛ Serving size= 1 cup, 189 (g); GI= 59 (Medium); GL= 9.2 (Low); Net carbs= 15.5 g

Watermelon ☛ Serving size= 1 cup, balls, 154 (g); GI= 72 (High); GL= 7.9 (Low); Net carbs= 11 g

GRAINS AND PASTA

Barley Cooked ☛ Serving size= 1 cup (170 g); GI= 25 (Low); GL= 10 (Low); Net carb= 40 g

Bulgur, Cooked ☛ Serving size= 1 cup (140 g); GI= 47 (Low); GL= 8.6 (Low); Net carb= 18.4 g

Chinese Chow Mein Noodles ☛ Serving size= 1/2 cup dry (28 g); GI= 35 (Low); GL= 5.6 (Low); Net carb= 15.9 g

Corn Bran Crude ☛ Serving size= 1 cup (76 g); GI= 75 (High); GL= 3.8 (Low); Net carb= 5 g

Hominy Canned Yellow ☛ Serving size= 1 cup (160 g); GI= 40 (Low); GL= 7.5 (Low); Net carb= 18.8 g

Japanese Somen Cooked ☛ Serving size= 2 oz (57 g); GI= 41 (Low); GL= 6.4 (Low); Net carb= 15.7 g

Noodles Cooked, made with Rice ☛ Serving size= 2 oz (57 g); GI= 56 (Medium); GL= 7.3 (Low); Net carb= 13.1 g

Pasta Cooked, Homemade, Prepared With Egg ☛ Serving size= 2 oz (57 g); GI= 66 (Medium); GL= 8.9 (Low); Net carb= 13.4 g

Pasta Cooked, Homemade, Prepared without Egg ☛ Serving size= 2 oz (57 g); GI= 66 (Medium); GL= 9.5 (Low); Net carb= 14.3 g

Pearled Barley Cooked ☛ Serving size= 1 cup (157 g); GI= 25 (Low); GL= 9.6 (Low); Net carb= 38.3 g

Spaghetti Cooked, Spinach ☛ Serving size= 2 oz (57 g); GI= 33 (Low); GL= 4.9 (Low); Net carb= 14.9 g

HERBS AND SPICES

Allspice ➥ Serving size= 1 tsp (2.1 g); GI= 15 (Low); GL= 0.3 (Low)

Basil ➥ Serving size= 1 tsp (0.7 g); GI= 70 (High); GL= 0 (Low)

Bay leaves ➥ Serving size= 1 tbsp, crumbled (1.8 g); GI= 23 (Low); GL= 0.1 (Low)

Black pepper ➥ Serving size= 1 tsp (2.4 g); GI= 44 (Low); GL= 0.3 (Low)

Cayenne pepper ➥ Serving size= 1 tsp (2.4 g); GI= 32 (Low); GL= 0.4 (Low)

Chiles ➥ Serving size= 1 tbsp (8 g); GI= 42 (Low); GL= 1.3 (Low)

Chives ➥ Serving size= 1 tbsp (2.8 g); GI= 15 (Low); GL= 0.3 (Low)

Cilantro ➥ Serving size= 1 cup (16 g); GI= 32 (Low); GL= 0 (Low)

Cinnamon ➥ Serving size= 1 tbsp (7.9 g); GI= 70 (High); GL= 2.1 (Low)

Coriander seed ➥ Serving size= 1 tbsp (5 g); GI= 33 (Low); GL= 1 (Low)

Cumin ☞ Serving size= 1 tbsp (6 g); GI= 0.0 (Low); GL= 0 (Low)

Curry powder ☞ Serving size= 1 tbsp (6 g); GI= 5 (Low); GL= 0.4 (Low)

Fennel seeds ☞ Serving size= 1 tbsp (5.8 g); GI= 16 (Low); GL= 0.3 (Low)

Ginger ☞ Serving size= 1 tsp (2.1 g); GI= 72 (High); GL= 0.3 (Low)

Mint ☞ Serving size= 1 tbsp (3.1 g) ; GI= 10 (Low); GL= 0.2 (Low)

Mustard Seed ☞ Serving size= 1 tsp (2 g); GI= 32 (Low); GL= 0.2 (Low)

Nutmeg ☞ Serving size= 1 tsp (2.4 g); GI= 46 (Low); GL= 0.3 (Low)

Oregano ☞ Serving size= 1 tbsp (3 g); GI= 5 (Low); GL= 0.3 (Low)

Paprika ☞ Serving size= 1 tsp (2 g); GI= 15 (Low); GL= 0.3 (Low)

Parsley ☞ Serving size= 1 tbsp (3 g); GI= 32 (Low); GL= 0.3 (Low)

Rosemary ☞ Serving size= 1 tbsp (3.3 g); GI= 70 (High); GL= 1.1 (Low)

Saffron ☞ Serving size= 1 tsp (0.7 g); GI= 70 (High); GL= 0.2 (Low)

Sesame seeds ☞ Serving size= 1 tbsp (10 g); GI= 31 (Low); GL= 0.1 (Low)

Thyme ☞ Serving size= 1 tbsp, leaves (2.7 g); GI= 51 (Low); GL= 0.1 (Low)

Turmeric ☞ Serving size= 1 tbsp (6.8 g); GI= 15 (Low); GL= 0.5 (Low)

Vanilla ☞ Serving size= 1 tbsp (4.4 g); GI= 16 (Low); GL= 0.5 (Low)

Wasabi powder ☞ Serving size= 1 tsp (2.8 g); GI= 31 (Low); GL= 0.3 (Low)

Wild garlic ☞ Serving size= 1 oz (28 g); GI= 11 (Low); GL= 2 (Low)

VEGETABLES

Alfalfa sprouts, raw ☞ GI= 32 (Low); Serving size= 1 cup (33 g); GL= 0.3 (Low); Net carb= 0.2 g

Algae, dried ☞ GI= 32 (Low); Serving size= 1 serv (7 g); GL= 1 (Low); Net carb= 0 g

Artichoke, Fresh, Frozen Or Canned, Cooked ☞ GI= 32 (Low); Serving size= 1 medium globe (103 g); GL= 1.4 (Low); Net carb= 4.5 g

Artichoke, Jerusalem, raw ☞ GI= 32 (Low); Serving size= 1 whole artichoke (173 g); GL= 2.4 (Low); Net carb= 7.6 g

Asparagus, Cooked, from Fresh, Frozen Or Canned ☞ GI= 32 (Low); Serving size= 8 spears (134 g); GL= 0.6 (Low); Net carb= 1.8 g

Asparagus, Raw ☞ GI= 28 (Low); Serving size= 8 spears (134 g); GL= 0.5 (Low); Net carb= 1.8 g

Bean sprouts, raw or cooked, from fresh or frozen ☞ GI= 32 (Low); Serving size= 1 cup (129 g); GL= 1.7 (Low); Net carb= 5.4 g

Beet greens, raw ☞ GI= 32 (Low); Serving size= 1 cup (124 g); GL= 1.7 (Low); Net carb= 5.4 g

Beets, raw or cooked, from fresh or frozen ☛ GI= 64 (Medium); Serving size= 1 cup, diced (157 g); GL= 8.2 (Low); Net carb= 12.8 g

Beets, pickled ☛ GI= 66 (Medium); Serving size= 1 cup, diced (157 g); GL= 8.4 (Low); Net carb= 12.8 g

Beets, raw ☛ GI= 64 (Medium); Serving size= 1 cup, diced (157 g); GL= 8.2 (Low); Net carb= 12.8 g

Broccoflower, Cooked ☛ GI= 32 (Low); Serving size= 1 cup (87 g); GL= 0.8 (Low); Net carb= 2.6 g

Broccoli, raw ☛ GI= 32 (Low); Serving size= 1 medium stalk (148 g); GL= 1.9 (Low); Net carb= 5.9 g

Brussels sprouts, raw ☛ GI= 32 (Low); Serving size= 1 cup (160 g); GL= 2.3 (Low); Net carb= 7.2 g

Cabbage, Chinese, cooked or raw ☛ GI= 32 (Low); Serving size= 1 cup, shredded (170 g); GL= 0.4 (Low); Net carb= 1.4 g

Cabbage, fresh or frozen, pickled, Japanese style ☛ GI= 32 (Low); Serving size= 1 cup (150 g); GL= 1.2 (Low); Net carb= 3.9 g

Cabbage, green, cooked ☛ GI= 32 (Low); Serving size= 1 cup (150 g); GL= 1.7 (Low); Net carb= 5.3 g

Cabbage, green, raw ☛ GI= 32 (Low); Serving size= 1 cup (150 g); GL= 1.7 (Low); Net carb= 5.3 g

Cabbage, red, cooked ☛ GI= 32 (Low); Serving size= 1 cup (150 g); GL= 1.7 (Low); Net carb= 5.3 g

Cabbage, red, pickled or raw ☛ GI= 32 (Low); Serving size= 1 cup (150 g); GL= 1.7 (Low); Net carb= 5.3 g

Cactus, Raw or Cooked ☛ GI= 7 (Low); Serving size= 1 cup (150 g); GL= 0.1 (Low); Net carb= 2 g

Calabaza (Spanish pumpkin), cooked ☛ GI= 75 (High); Serving size= 1 cup, cubes (166 g); GL= 6.2 (Low); Net carb= 8.3 g

Carrots, raw, cooked or canned ☛ GI= 47 (Low); Serving size= 1 cup or 1 carrot (151 g); GL= 4.8 (Low); Net carb= 10.2 g

Cauliflower, raw or pickled ☛ GI= 32 (Low); Serving size= 1 cup chopped (107 g); GL= 0.6 (Low); Net carb= 1.9 g

Celery juice ☛ GI= 32 (Low); Serving size= 1 cup (240 g); GL= 1.8 (Low); Net carb= 5.5 g

Celery, raw or cooked ☛ GI= 32 (Low); Serving size= 1 cup, diced (150 g); GL= 1.1 (Low); Net carb= 3.5 g

Chard, cooked ☛ GI= 32 (Low); Serving size= 1 cup, stalk and leaves (150 grams); GL= 1 (Low); Net carb= 3 g

Christophine, cooked ☛ GI= 32 (Low); Serving size= 1 cup (165 g); GL= 1.2 (Low); Net carb= 3.8 g

Coleslaw, with dressing ☛ GI= 44 (Low); Serving size= 1 cup (120 g); GL= 5.8 (Low); Net carb= 13.2 g

Collards, raw, or cooked, from fresh, frozen or canned ☛ GI= 32 (Low); Serving size= 1 cup, canned (170 g); GL= 2.3 (Low); Net carb= 7.3 g

Corn Cooked, From Fresh, Canned or Frozen ☛ GI= 48 (Low); Serving size= 1 cup (169 g); GL= 9.8 (Low); Net carb= 20.3 g

Corn Dried Cooked ☛ GI= 48 (Low); Serving size= 1 oz (28 g); GL= 1.8 (Low); Net carb= 3.8 g

Cucumber, raw or cooked ☛ GI= 32 (Low); Serving size= 1 cup (185 g); GL= 2.3 (Low); Net carb= 7.2 g

Cucumber, pickles, dill or fresh ☛ GI= 32 (Low); Serving size= 1 cup (185 g); GL= 2.3 (Low); Net carb= 7.2 g

Dandelion greens, raw ☛ GI= 32 (Low); Serving size= 1 cup (55 grams); GL= 0.6 (Low); Net carb= 1.9 g

Eggplant, cooked ☛ GI= 32 (Low); Serving size= 1 cup (1 inch cubes)

(99 g); GL= 1.8 (Low); Net carb= 5.6 g

Eggplant, pickled ☛ GI= 32 (Low); Serving size= 1 cup (155 g); GL= 2.8 (Low); Net carb= 8.7 g

Endive, raw ☛ GI= 32 (Low); Serving size= 1 cup, chopped (50 g); GL= 0.1 (Low); Net carb= 0.3 g

Fennel ☛ GI= 16 (Low); Serving size= 1 cup, sliced (87 g); GL= 0.6 (Low); Net carb= 3.7 g

Fennel Bulb, Cooked ☛ GI= 16 (Low); Serving size= 1 fennel bulb (218 g); GL= 2.3 (Low); Net carb= 14.1 g

Jicama, raw ☛ GI= 22 (Low); Serving size= 1 cup (130 g); GL= 1.5 (Low); Net carb= 6.6 g

Kale, raw ☛ GI= 32 (Low); Serving size= 1 cup 1 inch pieces (16 g); GL= 0 (Low); Net carb= 0.1 g

Kale, Cooked From Canned, Fresh or Frozen ☛ GI= 32 (Low); Serving size= 1 cup, chopped (130 g); GL= 1.2 (Low); Net carb= 3.9 g

Kohlrabi, raw ☛ GI= 21 (Low); Serving size= 1 cup (135 g); GL= 0.7 (Low); Net carb= 3.5 g

Kohlrabi, Cooked, Boiled Drained ☛ GI= 21 (Low); Serving size= 1 cup slices (165 g); GL= 1.9 (Low); Net carb= 9.2 g

Kohlrabi Creamed ☛ GI= 21 (Low); Serving size= 1 cup (187 g); GL= 2.8 (Low); Net carb= 13.2 g

Leeks, raw ☛ GI= 32 (Low); Serving size= 1 cup slices (165 g); GL= 6.5 (Low); Net carb= 20.4 g

Leeks, Cooked (Bulb And Lower Leaf-Portion) ☛ GI= 32 (Low); Serving size= 1 cup (170 g); GL= 3.6 (Low); Net carb= 11.3 g

Lettuce, arugula, raw ☛ GI= 32 (Low); Serving size= 1/6 medium head (89 g); GL= 0.7 (Low); Net carb= 2.3 g

Lettuce, Boston, raw ▶ GI= 32 (Low); Serving size= 1/6 medium head (89 g); GL= 0.7 (Low); Net carb= 2.3 g

Lettuce, raw or cooked ▶ GI= 32 (Low); Serving size= 1/6 medium head (89 g); GL= 0.7 (Low); Net carb= 2.3 g

Lotus Root, Cooked From Fresh, Frozen or Canned ▶ GI= 34 (Low); Serving size= 10 slices (81 g); GL= 3.4 (Low); Net carb= 10 g

Mushrooms, Cooked, From Canned, Fresh, or Frozen ▶ GI= 22 (Low); Serving size= 5 medium (89 g); GL= 0.5 (Low); Net carb= 2.3 g

Mushrooms, Creamed From Fresh, Frozen or Canned ▶ GI= 22 (Low); Serving size= 1 cup (217 g); GL= 2.6 (Low); Net carb= 11.9 g

Mushrooms Portobellos Grilled ▶ GI= 24 (Low); Serving size= 1 cup sliced (121 g); GL= 0.7 (Low); Net carb= 2.7 g

Mushrooms Shiitake, Cooked or Stir-Fried ▶ GI= 22 (Low); Serving size= 1 cup pieces (145 g); GL= 3.9 (Low); Net carb= 17.8 g

Mustard Cabbage, Cooked ▶ GI= 32 (Low); Serving size= 1 cup (175 g); GL= 0.4 (Low); Net carb= 1.3 g

Mustard Greens raw ▶ GI= 33 (Low); Serving size= 1 cup, chopped (56 g); GL= 0.3 (Low); Net carb= 0.8 g

Mustard Greens, Cooked From Fresh, Frozen or Canned ▶ GI= 33 (Low); Serving size= 1 cup, chopped (140 g); GL= 1.2 (Low); Net carb= 3.5 g

Mustard Spinach, raw or cooked (average) ▶ GI= 32 (Low); Serving size= 1 cup, chopped (150 g); GL= 0.5 (Low); Net carb= 1.7 g

New Zealand Spinach, Cooked ▶ GI= 33 (Low); Serving size= 1 cup, chopped (180 g); GL= 0.4 (Low); Net carb= 1.3 g

Nopales ▶ GI= 35 (Low); Serving size= 1 cup, sliced (86 g); GL= 0.3 (Low); Net carb= 1 g

Okra, Raw ☛ GI= 32 (Low); Serving size= 1 cup (100 g); GL= 1.4 (Low); Net carb= 4.3 g

Okra Cooked, From Fresh, Frozen or Canned ☛ GI= 32 (Low); Serving size= 1/2 cup slices (80 g); GL= 0.5 (Low); Net carb= 1.6 g

Onions, Raw ☛ GI= 15 (Low); Serving size= 1 cup, chopped (160 g); GL= 1.8 (Low); Net carb= 12.2 g

Onions Cooked, From Fresh, Frozen or Canned ☛ GI= 15 (Low); Serving size= 1 onion (63 g); GL= 0.3 (Low); Net carb= 1.8 g

Onions Dehydrated Flakes ☛ GI= 18 (Low); Serving size= 1 tbsp (5 g); GL= 0.7 (Low); Net carb= 3.7 g

Onions Creamed, From Fresh or Frozen ☛ GI= 15 (Low); Serving size= 1 cup (228 g); GL= 3 (Low); Net carb= 20 g

Onions Pearl Cooked, From Fresh, Frozen or Canned ☛ GI= 15 (Low); Serving size= 1 cup (185 g); GL= 2.4 (Low); Net carb= 16.1 g

Oriental Radishes ☛ GI= 32 (Low); Serving size= 1 cup slices (116 g); GL= 1.2 (Low); Net carb= 3.7 g

Palm Hearts, Canned ☛ GI= 38 (Low); Serving size= 1 cup (146 g); GL= 1.2 (Low); Net carb= 3.2 g

Parsnips ☛ GI= 48 (Low); Serving size= 1 cup slices (133 g); GL= 8.4 (Low); Net carb= 17.4 g

Parsnips, Cooked ☛ GI= 48 (Low); Serving size= 1/2 cup slices (78 g); GL= 4.9 (Low); Net carb= 10.1 g

Peas, green cooked, From Fresh, Frozen or Canned ☛ GI= 48 (Low); Serving size= 1 cup (175 g); GL= 8.3 (Low); Net carb= 17.3 g

Peas, green, raw ☛ GI= 48 (Low); Serving size= 1 cup (175 g); GL= 8.3 (Low); Net carb= 17.3 g

Pepper, hot chili, raw ☛ GI= 32 (Low); Serving size= 1 pepper (73 g); GL= 0.9 (Low); Net carb= 2.8 g

Pepper hot cooked, from Fresh, Frozen or canned ☛ GI= 32 (Low); Serving size= 1 pepper (73 g); GL= 0.9 (Low); Net carb= 2.8 g

Pepper, hot, pickled ☛ GI= 32 (Low); Serving size= 1 pepper (73 g); GL= 0.9 (Low); Net carb= 2.8 g

Pepper, pickled ☛ GI= 32 (Low); Serving size= 1 pepper (73 g); GL= 0.9 (Low); Net carb= 2.8 g

Pepper, poblano, raw ☛ GI= 32 (Low); Serving size= 1 pepper (73 g); GL= 0.9 (Low); Net carb= 2.8 g

Pepper, Serrano, raw ☛ GI= 32 (Low); Serving size= 1 cup (110 g); GL= 4.2 (Low); Net carb= 13.2 g

Pepper, sweet, green, raw ☛ GI= 32 (Low); Serving size= 1 cup (110 g); GL= 4.1 (Low); Net carb= 12.9 g

Pepper, sweet, red, raw ☛ GI= 32 (Low); Serving size= 1 cup (110 g); GL= 4.2 (Low); Net carb= 13 g

Pimiento ☛ GI= 32 (Low); Serving size= 1 cup (185 g); GL= 4.7 (Low); Net carb= 14.8 g

Radish, common, raw ☛ GI= 32 (Low); Serving size= 1 cup slices (116 g); GL= 1.9 (Low); Net carb= 5.9 g

Romaine Lettuce ☛ GI= 32 (Low); Serving size= 1 cup shredded (47 g); GL= 0.2 (Low); Net carb= 0.6 g

Rutabaga Cooked ☛ GI= 72 (High); Serving size= 1 cup, pieces (175 g); GL= 6.2 (Low); Net carb= 8.6 g

Salsify, Raw ☛ GI= 30 (Low); Serving size= 1 cup slices (133 g); GL= 6.1 (Low); Net carb= 20.3 g

Salsify Cooked, From Fresh, Frozen or Canned ☛ GI= 30 (Low); Serving size= 1 cup slices (135 g); GL= 5 (Low); Net carb= 16.6 g

Sauerkraut ☛ GI= 32 (Low); Serving size= 1 cup (142 g); GL= 0.6 (Low); Net carb= 2 g

Sauerkraut Cooked, From Fresh, Frozen or canned ☞ GI= 32 (Low); Serving size= 1 cup (142 g); GL= 0.7 (Low); Net carb= 2.1 g

Savoy Cabbage ☞ GI= 32 (Low); Serving size= 1 cup, shredded (70 g); GL= 0.7 (Low); Net carb= 2.1 g

Scallop Squash ☞ GI= 48 (Low); Serving size= 1 cup slices (130 g); GL= 1.6 (Low); Net carb= 3.4 g

Seaweed Agar Raw ☞ GI= 48 (Low); Serving size= 2 tbsp (1/8 cup) (10 g); GL= 0.3 (Low); Net carb= 0.6 g

Snow Peas Cooked, From Fresh, Frozen or Canned ☞ GI= 30 (Low); Serving size= 1 cup, chopped (98 g); GL= 1.5 (Low); Net carb= 4.9 g

Soybean Sprouts ☞ GI= 15 (Low); Serving size= 1/2 cup (35 g); GL= 0.4 (Low); Net carb= 3 g

Soybeans Green Cooked ☞ GI= 15 (Low); Serving size= 1 cup (180 g); GL= 1.8 (Low); Net carb= 12.3 g

Soybeans Mature Seeds Cooked ☞ GI= 15 (Low); Serving size= 1 cup (94 g); GL= 0.8 (Low); Net carb= 5.4 g

Spinach Cooked, From Fresh, Frozen or Canned ☞ GI= 18 (Low); Serving size= 1 cup (30 g); GL= 0.1 (Low); Net carb= 0.4 g

Spring Onions ☞ GI= 15 (Low); Serving size= 1 cup, chopped (100 g); GL= 0.7 (Low); Net carb= 4.7 g

Squash Spaghetti, Raw ☞ GI= 20 (Low); Serving size= 1 cup, cubes (101 g); GL= 1.1 (Low); Net carb= 5.4 g

Squash Spaghetti, Cooked ☞ GI= 20 (Low); Serving size= 1 cup, cooked, (160 g); GL= 1.5 (Low); Net carb= 7.7 g

Squash Summer ☞ GI= 15 (Low); Serving size= 1 cup (217 g); GL= 1.7 (Low); Net carb= 11.6 g

Squash Winter, Cooked ☞ GI= 15 (Low); Serving size= 1 cup, cubes (205 g); GL= 1.9 (Low); Net carb= 12.4 g

Sun-Dried Tomatoes ☞ GI= 36 (Low); Serving size= 1 cup (54 g); GL= 8.4 (Low); Net carb= 23.5 g

Swamp Cabbage ☞ GI= 32 (Low); Serving size= 1 cup, chopped (56 g); GL= 0.2 (Low); Net carb= 0.6 g

Swamp Cabbage Cooked ☞ GI= 32 (Low); Serving size= 1 cup, chopped (98 g); GL= 0.6 (Low); Net carb= 1.8 g

Sweet Potato Cooked, Boiled ☞ GI= 66 (Medium); Serving size= 1 small (80 g); GL= 7.6 (Low); Net carb= 11.5 g

Swiss Chard ☞ GI= 32 (Low); Serving size= 1 cup (36 g); GL= 0.2 (Low); Net carb= 0.8 g

Taro ☞ GI= 32 (Low); Serving size= 1 cup, sliced (104 g); GL= 7.4 (Low); Net carb= 23.3 g

Taro Leaves Cooked ☞ GI= 32 (Low); Serving size= 1 cup (145 g); GL= 0.9 (Low); Net carb= 2.7 g

Taro Leaves Raw ☞ GI= 32 (Low); Serving size= 1 cup (28 g); GL= 0.3 (Low); Net carb= 0.8 g

Tomatillos ☞ GI= 38 (Low); Serving size= 1 medium (34 g); GL= 0.5 (Low); Net carb= 1.3 g

Tomatoes ☞ GI= 38 (Low); Serving size= 1 cup cherry tomatoes (149 g); GL= 1.5 (Low); Net carb= 4 g

Tomatoes, Cooked, From Fresh, Frozen or Canned ☞ GI= 38 (Low); Serving size= 1 cup (240 g); GL= 3 (Low); Net carb= 7.9 g

Tomatoes Crushed Canned ☞ GI= 38 (Low); Serving size= 1/2 cup (121 g); GL= 2.5 (Low); Net carb= 6.5 g

Sun-Dried Tomatoes Packed In Oil ☞ GI= 38 (Low); Serving size= 1 cup (110 g); GL= 7.3 (Low); Net carb= 19.3 g

Turnip Cooked, From Fresh, Frozen or Canned ☞ GI= 32 (Low); Serving size= 1 cup, pieces (155 g); GL= 1.5 (Low); Net carb= 4.7 g

Turnip Greens ⮕ GI= 32 (Low); Serving size= 1 cup, chopped (55 g); GL= 0.7 (Low); Net carb= 2.2 g

Wakame ⮕ GI= 50 (Low); Serving size= 2 tbsp (1/8 cup) (10 g); GL= 0.4 (Low); Net carb= 0.9 g

Wasabi Root ⮕ GI= 41 (Low); Serving size= 1 cup, sliced (130 g); GL= 8.4 (Low); Net carb= 20.5 g

Waterchestnuts Chinese Raw or Canned ⮕ GI= 54 (Low); Serving size= 1/2 cup slices (62 g); GL= 7 (Low); Net carb= 13 g

Watercress ⮕ GI= 32 (Low); Serving size= 1 cup, chopped (34 g); GL= 0.1 (Low); Net carb= 0.3 g

Watercress, Cooked ⮕ GI= 32 (Low); Serving size= 1 cup (142 g); GL= 0.3 (Low); Net carb= 1 g

Winged Bean Immature Seeds, Cooked ⮕ GI= 50 (Low); Serving size= 1 cup (62 g); GL= 1 (Low); Net carb= 2 g

Winged Beans Immature Seeds Raw ⮕ GI= 50 (Low); Serving size= 1 cup slices (44 g); GL= 0.9 (Low); Net carb= 1.9 g

Winter Squash ⮕ GI= 51 (Low); Serving size= 1 cup, cubes (116 g); GL= 4.2 (Low); Net carb= 8.2 g

Yardlong Bean Cooked ⮕ GI= 82 (High); Serving size= 1 cup slices (104 g); GL= 7.8 (Low); Net carb= 9.5 g

Yardlong Bean Raw ⮕ GI= 82 (High); Serving size= 1 cup slices (91 g); GL= 6.2 (Low); Net carb= 7.6 g

Zucchini ⮕ GI= 15 (Low); Serving size= 1 cup, chopped (124 g); GL= 0.4 (Low); Net carb= 2.6 g

PART VII
THE WORST FOODS TO EAT (HIGH GLYCEMIC LOAD FOOD)

❄

BAKED PRODUCTS

Basbousa ☞ Serving size= 1 piece (about 3 x 2-1/2 inch), 82 g; GI= 63 (Medium); GL= 25.5 (High); Net carb= 40.5 g

Biscuit—Plain Or Buttermilk Dry Mix ☞ Serving size= 1 cup, purchased, 120 g; GI= 70 (High); GL= 51.5 (High); Net carb= 73.6 g

Bread—Chapati Or Roti Plain ☞ Serving size= 1 piece, 68 g; GI= 81 (High); GL= 22.8 (High); Net carb= 28.2 g

Bread—French Or Vienna Whole Wheat ☞ Serving size= 1 slice 1 serving, 48 g; GI= 95 (High); GL= 20.5 (High); Net carb= 21.6 g

Brioche ☞ Serving size= 1 piece, 77 g; GI= 91 (High); GL= 24.1 (High); Net carb= 26.5 g

Cupcake, German Chocolate ☞ Serving size= 1 regular cupcake, 75 g; GI= 55 (Medium); GL= 20.1 (High); Net carb= 36.6 g

Cupcake, Fruit ☞ Serving size= 1 regular cupcake, 75 g; GI= 55 (Medium); GL= 22.6 (High); Net carb= 41 g

Cupcake, Nut ☞ Serving size= 1 regular cupcake, 75 g; GI= 55 (Medium); GL= 21.8 (High); Net carb= 39.7 g

Cake, White, Made From Recipe ☛ Serving size= 1 piece, 74 g; GI= 55 (Medium); GL= 22.9 (High); Net carb= 41.7 g

Cake, Yellow Enriched Dry Mix ☛ Serving size= 1 serving, 43 g; GI= 55 (Medium); GL= 19.1 (High); Net carb= 34.7 g

Cake, Yellow, Made From Recipe ☛ Serving size= 1 piece, 68 g; GI= 55 (Medium); GL= 19.6 (High); Net carb= 35.6 g

Cobbler, Apple ☛ Serving size= 1 cup, 217 g; GI= 67 (Medium); GL= 51.7 (High); Net carb= 77.2 g

Cobbler, Apricot ☛ Serving size= 1 cup, 217 g; GI= 67 (Medium); GL= 49.4 (High); Net carb= 73.7 g

Cobbler, Berry ☛ Serving size= 1 cup, 217 g; GI= 67 (Medium); GL= 60 (High); Net carb= 89.5 g

Cobbler, Cherry ☛ Serving size= 1 cup, 217 g; GI= 67 (Medium); GL= 50.3 (High); Net carb= 75.1 g

Cobbler, Peach ☛ Serving size= 1 cup, 217 g; GI= 67 (Medium); GL= 53.4 (High); Net carb= 79.7 g

Cobbler, Pear ☛ Serving size= 1 cup, 217 g; GI= 67 (Medium); GL= 57.8 (High); Net carb= 86.2 g

Cobbler, Pineapple ☛ Serving size= 1 cup, 217 g; GI= 67 (Medium); GL= 52.3 (High); Net carb= 78 g

Cobbler, Plum ☛ Serving size= 1 cup, 217 g; GI= 67 (Medium); GL= 53.9 (High); Net carb= 80.4 g

Cobbler, Rhubarb ☛ Serving size= 1 cup, 217 g; GI= 67 (Medium); GL= 66.3 (High); Net carb= 98.9 g

CornBread, Muffin, Round, Home Recipe ☛ Serving size= 1 small, 66 g; GI= 73 (High); GL= 21.3 (High); Net carb= 29.2 g

Cornmeal, Dumpling ☛ Serving size= 1 cup, cooked, 240 g; GI= 75 (High); GL= 43.7 (High); Net carb= 58.3 g

Cream Puff Eclair Custard ☛ Serving size= 4 oz, 113 g; GI= 59 (Medium); GL= 24.4 (High); Net carb= 41.3 g

Crisp Apple Apple Dessert ☛ Serving size= 1 cup, 246 g; GI= 61 (Medium); GL= 43.8 (High); Net carb= 71.8 g

Crisp Blueberry ☛ Serving size= 1 cup, 246 g; GI= 59 (Medium); GL= 57 (High); Net carb= 96.6 g

Crisp Cherry ☛ Serving size= 1 cup, 246 g; GI= 60 (Medium); GL= 68.2 (High); Net carb= 113.6 g

Crisp Peach ☛ Serving size= 1 cup, 246 g; GI= 63 (Medium); GL= 56.6 (High); Net carb= 89.8 g

Crisp Rhubarb ☛ Serving size= 1 cup, 246 g; GI= 59 (Medium); GL= 59.9 (High); Net carb= 101.5 g

Doughnut, Chocolate Cream-Filled ☛ Serving size= 1 doughnut, 65 g; GI= 75 (High); GL= 19.4 (High); Net carb= 25.9 g

Doughnut, Chocolate, With Chocolate Icing ☛ Serving size= 1 doughnut (3 inch dia), 71 g; GI= 78 (High); GL= 27.9 (High); Net carb= 35.8 g

Doughnut, Custard-Filled With Icing ☛ Serving size= 1 doughnut, 70 g; GI= 79 (High); GL= 30 (High); Net carb= 38 g

Doughnut, Chocolate Covered, Raised Or Yeast ☛ Serving size= 1 doughnut (3 inch dia), 71 g; GI= 77 (High); GL= 27.5 (High); Net carb= 35.7 g

Dutch Apple Pie ☛ Serving size= 1/8 pie 1 pie (1/8 of 9 inch pie), 131 g; GI= 55 (Medium); GL= 31 (High); Net carb= 56.3 g

English Muffins, Whole Grain White ☛ Serving size= 1 muffin 1 serving, 57 g; GI= 77 (High); GL= 20.5 (High); Net carb= 26.6 g

Muffin, Chocolate Chip ☛ Serving size= 1 muffin, 58 g; GI= 63 (Medium); GL= 19.5 (High); Net carb= 31 g

Muffin, English Oat Bran With Raisins ☛ Serving size= 1 muffin, 58 g; GI= 70 (High); GL= 19.3 (High); Net carb= 27.6 g

Pie Crust, Cookie-Type Chocolate ☛ Serving size= 1 crust, 182 g; GI= 59 (Medium); GL= 66.3 (High); Net carb= 112.4 g

Pie Crust, Cookie-Type, Vanilla Wafer Chilled ☛ Serving size= 1 cup, 129 g; GI= 59 (Medium); GL= 38.1 (High); Net carb= 64.6 g

Pie Crust, Refrigerated Regular Baked ☛ Serving size= 1 pie crust, 198 g; GI= 59 (Medium); GL= 66.7 (High); Net carb= 113.1 g

Pie, Apple Diet ☛ Serving size= 1 individual serving, 85 g; GI= 59 (Medium); GL= 21.4 (High); Net carb= 36.2 g

Pie, Banana Cream Individual Size Or Tart ☛ Serving size= 1 tart, 117 g; GI= 59 (Medium); GL= 20.7 (High); Net carb= 35 g

Pie, Berry, Individual Size Or Tart ☛ Serving size= 1 tart, 117 g; GI= 59 (Medium); GL= 26.6 (High); Net carb= 45.1 g

Pie—Blackberry Individual Size Or Tart ☛ Serving size= 1 tart, 117 g; GI= 59 (Medium); GL= 23.4 (High); Net carb= 39.7 g

Pie, Blueberry Tart ☛ Serving size= 1 tart, 117 g; GI= 59 (Medium); GL= 25.5 (High); Net carb= 43.3 g

Pie, Chocolate Cream Tart ☛ Serving size= 1 tart, 117 g; GI= 59 (Medium); GL= 24 (High); Net carb= 40.6 g

Pie, Chocolate Creme, Commercially Prepared ☛ Serving size= 1 serving .167 pie, 120 g; GI= 59 (Medium); GL= 26.7 (High); Net carb= 45.2 g

Pie, Peach Tart ☛ Serving size= 1 tart, 117 g; GI= 59 (Medium); GL= 26 (High); Net carb= 44.1 g

Pie—Pear Individual Size Or Tart ☛ Serving size= 1 tart, 117 g; GI= 59 (Medium); GL= 25.6 (High); Net carb= 43.4 g

Pie, Pudding Chocolate ☞ Serving size= 1 individual pie, 142 g; GI= 59 (Medium); GL= 34.3 (High); Net carb= 58.2 g

Pie, Pudding Flavors, Tart, Other Than Chocolate ☞ Serving size= 1 small tart, 117 g; GI= 59 (Medium); GL= 26.1 (High); Net carb= 44.3 g

Pie, Raisin Tart ☞ Serving size= 1 tart, 117 g; GI= 59 (Medium); GL= 27 (High); Net carb= 45.8 g

Pie, Rhubarb, Tart ☞ Serving size= 1 tart, 117 g; GI= 59 (Medium); GL= 25.1 (High); Net carb= 42.5 g

Pie, Strawberry Cream Tart ☞ Serving size= 1 tart, 117 g; GI= 59 (Medium); GL= 19.1 (High); Net carb= 32.3 g

Pie, Strawberry Tart ☞ Serving size= 1 tart, 117 g; GI= 59 (Medium); GL= 23.9 (High); Net carb= 40.5 g

Pizza Gluten-Free, Cheese And Vegetables, Thick Crust ☞ Serving size= 1 piece, 149 g; GI= 61 (Medium); GL= 21.4 (High); Net carb= 35.1 g

Pizza, Whole Wheat, Cheese And Vegetables, Thick Crust ☞ Serving size= 1 piece, nfs, 149 g; GI= 62 (Medium); GL= 23.2 (High); Net carb= 37.4 g

Pizza, Cheese From School Lunch (Medium Crust) ☞ Serving size= 1 piece, 147 g; GI= 63 (Medium); GL= 24.4 (High); Net carb= 38.7 g

Pizza Gluten-Free, Cheese, Thick Crust ☞ Serving size= 1 piece, 132 g; GI= 63 (Medium); GL= 22.6 (High); Net carb= 35.8 g

Pizza, Whole Wheat, Cheese, Thick Crust ☞ Serving size= 1 piece, 132 g; GI= 64 (Medium); GL= 24.5 (High); Net carb= 38.3 g

Pizza, Cheese With Fruit Medium Crust ☞ Serving size= 1 piece, 137 g; GI= 64 (Medium); GL= 25.3 (High); Net carb= 39.5 g

Pizza, Cheese With Fruit, Thick Crust ☞ Serving size= 1 piece, nfs, 150 g; GI= 64 (Medium); GL= 27.8 (High); Net carb= 43.4 g

Pizza, Frozen, Cheese With Vegetables, Thick Crust ☛ Serving size= 1 piece, 143 g; GI= 64 (Medium); GL= 26.4 (High); Net carb= 41.3 g

Pizza, From Restaurant Or Fast Food, Cheese With Vegetables, Medium Crust ☛ Serving size= 1 piece, 133 g; GI= 64 (Medium); GL= 24.3 (High); Net carb= 37.9 g

Pizza—Cheese With Vegetables From Restaurant Or Fast Food—Thick Crust ☛ Serving size= 1 piece, nfs, 149 g; GI= 64 (Medium); GL= 27 (High); Net carb= 42.2 g

Pizza, Extra Cheese, Thick Crust ☛ Serving size= 1 piece, nfs, 141 g; GI= 65 (Medium); GL= 27.3 (High); Net carb= 42 g

Pizza, Without Cheese, Thick Crust ☛ Serving size= 1 piece, nfs, 124 g; GI= 73 (High); GL= 32.5 (High); Net carb= 44.5 g

Pizza Rolls ☛ Serving size= 1 cup, 119 g; GI= 80 (High); GL= 49.6 (High); Net carb= 62 g

Roll Sweet Frosted ☛ Serving size= 1 small, 54 g; GI= 77 (High); GL= 20.1 (High); Net carb= 26.1 g

Roll Sweet With Fruit Frosted ☛ Serving size= 1 small, 54 g; GI= 77 (High); GL= 21.4 (High); Net carb= 27.8 g

Waffle Chocolate Chip Frozen—Ready-To-Heat ☛ Serving size= 2 waffles, 70 g; GI= 76 (High); GL= 23.5 (High); Net carb= 30.9 g

Waffle Whole Wheat Low-fat Frozen—Ready-To-Heat ☛ Serving size= 1 serving 2 waffles, 70 g; GI= 72 (High); GL= 22.6 (High); Net carb= 31.4 g

BEEF, LAMP, VEAL, PORK & POULTRY

❄

Beef-Offal—Heart: Breaded + fried ☞ Serving size= 3 oz, 85 g; GI= 95 (High); GL= 20 (High); Net carb= 21 g

Beef—Bottom Round: Breaded + fried ☞ Serving size= 3 oz, 85 g; GI= 95 (High); GL= 20 (High); Net carb= 21 g

Beef—Brain: Breaded + fried ☞ Serving size= 3 oz, 85 g; GI= 95 (High); GL= 20 (High); Net carb= 21 g

Beef—Brisket: Breaded + fried ☞ Serving size= 3 oz, 85 g; GI= 95 (High); GL= 20 (High); Net carb= 21 g

Beef—Chuck Roast: Breaded + fried ☞ Serving size= 3 oz, 85 g; GI= 95 (High); GL= 20 (High); Net carb= 21 g

Beef—Chuck Steak Varieties Chart: Breaded + fried ☞ Serving size= 3 oz, 85 g; GI= 95 (High); GL= 20 (High); Net carb= 21 g

Beef—Cuts of Steak: Breaded + fried ☞ Serving size= 3 oz, 85 g; GI= 95 (High); GL= 20 (High); Net carb= 21 g

Beef—Delmonico Steak: Breaded + fried ☞ Serving size= 3 oz, 85 g; GI= 95 (High); GL= 20 (High); Net carb= 21 g

Beef—Hanger Steak: Breaded + fried ➨ Serving size= 3 oz, 85 g; GI= 95 (High); GL= 20 (High); Net carb= 21 g

Beef—Kidney: Breaded + fried ➨ Serving size= 1 slice, 81 g; GI= 95 (High); GL= 20 (High); Net carb= 21 g

Beef—Liver: Battered + fried ➨ Serving size= 1 slice, 81 g; GI= 95 (High); GL= 20 (High); Net carb= 21.1 g

Beef—Liver: Breaded + fried ➨ Serving size= 1 slice, 81 g; GI= 95 (High); GL= 23.8 (High); Net carb= 25.1 g

Beef—Loin Steaks and/or Steak Types: Breaded + fried ➨ Serving size= 3 oz, 85 g; GI= 95 (High); GL= 20 (High); Net carb= 21 g

Beef—Mock Tender Petite Fillet: Breaded + fried ➨ Serving size= 3 oz, 85 g; GI= 95 (High); GL= 20 (High); Net carb= 21 g

Beef—Prime Rib: Breaded + fried ➨ Serving size= 3 oz, 85 g; GI= 95 (High); GL= 20 (High); Net carb= 21 g

Beef—Rib Steak Cuts: Breaded + fried ➨ Serving size= 3 oz, 85 g; GI= 95 (High); GL= 20 (High); Net carb= 21 g

Beef—Round Steak Varieties: Breaded + fried ➨ Serving size= 3 oz, 85 g; GI= 95 (High); GL= 20 (High); Net carb= 21 g

Beef—Short Loin: Breaded + fried ➨ Serving size= 3 oz, 85 g; GI= 95 (High); GL= 20 (High); Net carb= 21 g

Beef—Short Ribs: Breaded + fried ➨ Serving size= 3 oz, 85 g; GI= 95 (High); GL= 20 (High); Net carb= 21 g

Beef—T-Bone Steak: Breaded + fried ➨ Serving size= 3 oz, 85 g; GI= 95 (High); GL= 20 (High); Net carb= 21 g

Beef—Tenderloin: Breaded + fried ➨ Serving size= 3 oz, 85 g; GI= 95 (High); GL= 20 (High); Net carb= 21 g

Beef—Tongue: Breaded + fried ➨ Serving size= 1 slice, 81 g; GI= 95 (High); GL= 20 (High); Net carb= 21 g

Beef—Top Sirloin: Breaded + fried ☛ Serving size= 3 oz, 85 g; GI= 95 (High); GL= 20 (High); Net carb= 21 g

Beef—Tri-Tip: Breaded + fried ☛ Serving size= 3 oz, 85 g; GI= 95 (High); GL= 20 (High); Net carb= 21 g

Beef—Tripe: Breaded + fried ☛ Serving size= 1 slice, 81 g; GI= 95 (High); GL= 20 (High); Net carb= 21 g

Chicken—Backs and Necks: Breaded + fried ☛ Serving size= 3 oz, 85 g; GI= 95 (High); GL= 20 (High); Net carb= 21 g

Chicken—Breast Fillet Tenderloin: Breaded + fried ☛ Serving size= 3 oz, 85 g; GI= 95 (High); GL= 20 (High); Net carb= 21 g

Chicken—Drumstick: Breaded + fried ☛ Serving size= 3 oz, 85 g; GI= 95 (High); GL= 20 (High); Net carb= 21 g

Chicken—Leg: Breaded + fried ☛ Serving size= 3 oz, 85 g; GI= 95 (High); GL= 20 (High); Net carb= 21 g

Chicken—Tender: Breaded + fried ☛ Serving size= 3 oz, 85 g; GI= 95 (High); GL= 20 (High); Net carb= 21 g

Chicken—Thigh: Breaded + fried ☛ Serving size= 3 oz, 85 g; GI= 95 (High); GL= 20 (High); Net carb= 21 g

Chicken—Wing: Breaded + fried ☛ Serving size= 3 oz, 85 g; GI= 95 (High); GL= 20 (High); Net carb= 21 g

Lamb—Breast: Breaded + fried ☛ Serving size= 3 oz, 85 g; GI= 95 (High); GL= 20 (High); Net carb= 21 g

Lamb—Cutlets: Breaded + fried ☛ Serving size= 3 oz, 85 g; GI= 95 (High); GL= 20 (High); Net carb= 21 g

Lamb—Leg: Breaded + fried ☛ Serving size= 3 oz, 85 g; GI= 95 (High); GL= 20 (High); Net carb= 21 g

Lamb—Loin: Breaded + fried ☛ Serving size= 3 oz, 85 g; GI= 95 (High); GL= 20 (High); Net carb= 21 g

Lamb—Neck: Breaded + fried ☞ Serving size= 3 oz, 85 g; GI= 95 (High); GL= 20 (High); Net carb= 21 g

Lamb—Rack: Breaded + fried ☞ Serving size= 3 oz, 85 g; GI= 95 (High); GL= 20 (High); Net carb= 21 g

Lamb—Rump: Breaded + fried ☞ Serving size= 3 oz, 85 g; GI= 95 (High); GL= 20 (High); Net carb= 21 g

Lamb—Shank: Breaded + fried ☞ Serving size= 3 oz, 85 g; GI= 95 (High); GL= 20 (High); Net carb= 21 g

Lamb—Shoulder: Breaded + fried ☞ Serving size= 3 oz, 85 g; GI= 95 (High); GL= 20 (High); Net carb= 21 g

Pork—back ribs: Breaded + fried ☞ Serving size= 3 oz, 85 g; GI= 95 (High); GL= 20 (High); Net carb= 21 g

Pork—Belly: Breaded + fried ☞ Serving size= 3 oz, 85 g; GI= 95 (High); GL= 20 (High); Net carb= 21 g

Pork—Cutlets: Breaded + fried ☞ Serving size= 3 oz, 85 g; GI= 95 (High); GL= 20 (High); Net carb= 21 g

Pork—Garlic Sausages: Breaded + fried ☞ Serving size= 3 oz, 85 g; GI= 95 (High); GL= 20 (High); Net carb= 21 g

Pork—Ham: Breaded + fried ☞ Serving size= 3 oz, 85 g; GI= 95 (High); GL= 20 (High); Net carb= 21 g

Pork—Loin: Breaded + fried ☞ Serving size= 3 oz, 85 g; GI= 95 (High); GL= 20 (High); Net carb= 21 g

Pork—Rib chops: Breaded + fried ☞ Serving size= 3 oz, 85 g; GI= 95 (High); GL= 20 (High); Net carb= 21 g

Pork—Roasts: Breaded + fried ☞ Serving size= 3 oz, 85 g; GI= 95 (High); GL= 20 (High); Net carb= 21 g

Pork—Sausages: Breaded + fried ☞ Serving size= 3 oz, 85 g; GI= 95 (High); GL= 20 (High); Net carb= 21 g

Pork—Shoulder chops: Breaded + fried ☞ Serving size= 3 oz, 85 g; GI= 95 (High); GL= 20 (High); Net carb= 21 g

Pork—Sirloin chops: Breaded + fried ☞ Serving size= 3 oz, 85 g; GI= 95 (High); GL= 20 (High); Net carb= 21 g

Pork—spare ribs: Breaded + fried ☞ Serving size= 3 oz, 85 g; GI= 95 (High); GL= 20 (High); Net carb= 21 g

Turkey—Backs and Necks: Breaded + fried ☞ Serving size= 3 oz, 85 g; GI= 95 (High); GL= 20 (High); Net carb= 21 g

Turkey—Breast Fillet Tenderloin: Breaded + fried ☞ Serving size= 3 oz, 85 g; GI= 95 (High); GL= 20 (High); Net carb= 21 g

Turkey—Breast: Breaded + fried ☞ Serving size= 3 oz, 85 g; GI= 95 (High); GL= 20 (High); Net carb= 21 g

Turkey—Drumstick: Breaded + fried ☞ Serving size= 3 oz, 85 g; GI= 95 (High); GL= 20 (High); Net carb= 21 g

Turkey—Leg: Breaded + fried ☞ Serving size= 3 oz, 85 g; GI= 95 (High); GL= 20 (High); Net carb= 21 g

Turkey—Tender: Breaded + fried ☞ Serving size= 3 oz, 85 g; GI= 95 (High); GL= 20 (High); Net carb= 21 g

Turkey—Thigh: Breaded + fried ☞ Serving size= 3 oz, 85 g; GI= 95 (High); GL= 20 (High); Net carb= 21 g

Turkey—Wing: Breaded + fried ☞ Serving size= 3 oz, 85 g; GI= 95 (High); GL= 20 (High); Net carb= 21 g

Veal-Offal—Heart: Breaded + fried ☞ Serving size= 3 oz, 85 g; GI= 95 (High); GL= 20 (High); Net carb= 21 g

Veal—Bottom Round: Breaded + fried ☞ Serving size= 3 oz, 85 g; GI= 95 (High); GL= 20 (High); Net carb= 21 g

Veal—Brain: Breaded + fried ☞ Serving size= 3 oz, 85 g; GI= 95 (High); GL= 20 (High); Net carb= 21 g

Veal—Brisket: Breaded + fried ☞ Serving size= 3 oz, 85 g; GI= 95 (High); GL= 20 (High); Net carb= 21 g

Veal—Chuck Roast: Breaded + fried ☞ Serving size= 3 oz, 85 g; GI= 95 (High); GL= 20 (High); Net carb= 21 g

Veal—Chuck Steak Varieties Chart: Breaded + fried ☞ Serving size= 3 oz, 85 g; GI= 95 (High); GL= 20 (High); Net carb= 21 g

Veal—Cuts of Steak: Breaded + fried ☞ Serving size= 3 oz, 85 g; GI= 95 (High); GL= 20 (High); Net carb= 21 g

Veal—Delmonico Steak: Breaded + fried ☞ Serving size= 3 oz, 85 g; GI= 95 (High); GL= 20 (High); Net carb= 21 g

Veal—Hanger Steak: Breaded + fried ☞ Serving size= 3 oz, 85 g; GI= 95 (High); GL= 20 (High); Net carb= 21 g

Veal—Kidney: Breaded + fried ☞ Serving size= 2 slice, 81 g; GI= 95 (High); GL= 20 (High); Net carb= 21 g

Veal—Liver: Battered + fried ☞ Serving size= 1 slice, 81 g; GI= 95 (High); GL= 20 (High); Net carb= 21.1 g

Veal—Liver: Breaded + fried ☞ Serving size= 1 slice, 81 g; GI= 95 (High); GL= 23.8 (High); Net carb= 25.1 g

Veal—Loin Steaks and/or Steak Types: Breaded + fried ☞ Serving size= 3 oz, 85 g; GI= 95 (High); GL= 20 (High); Net carb= 21 g

Veal—Mock Tender Petite Fillet: Breaded + fried ☞ Serving size= 3 oz, 85 g; GI= 95 (High); GL= 20 (High); Net carb= 21 g

Veal—Prime Rib: Breaded + fried ☞ Serving size= 3 oz, 85 g; GI= 95 (High); GL= 20 (High); Net carb= 21 g

Veal—Rib Steak Cuts: Breaded + fried ☞ Serving size= 3 oz, 85 g; GI= 95 (High); GL= 20 (High); Net carb= 21 g

Veal—Round Steak Varieties: Breaded + fried ☞ Serving size= 3 oz, 85 g; GI= 95 (High); GL= 20 (High); Net carb= 21 g

Veal—Short Loin: Breaded + fried ☛ Serving size= 3 oz, 85 g; GI= 95 (High); GL= 20 (High); Net carb= 21 g

Veal—Short Ribs: Breaded + fried ☛ Serving size= 3 oz, 85 g; GI= 95 (High); GL= 20 (High); Net carb= 21 g

Veal—T-Bone Steak: Breaded + fried ☛ Serving size= 3 oz, 85 g; GI= 95 (High); GL= 20 (High); Net carb= 21 g

Veal—Tenderloin: Breaded + fried ☛ Serving size= 3 oz, 85 g; GI= 95 (High); GL= 20 (High); Net carb= 21 g

Veal—Tongue: Breaded + fried ☛ Serving size= 1 slice, 81 g; GI= 95 (High); GL= 20 (High); Net carb= 21 g

Veal—Top Sirloin: Breaded + fried ☛ Serving size= 3 oz, 85 g; GI= 95 (High); GL= 20 (High); Net carb= 21 g

Veal—Tri-Tip: Breaded + fried ☛ Serving size= 3 oz, 85 g; GI= 95 (High); GL= 20 (High); Net carb= 21 g

Veal—Tripe: Breaded + fried ☛ Serving size= 3 oz, 85 g; GI= 95 (High); GL= 20 (High); Net carb= 21 g

BEVERAGES

— **People with diabetes must avoid heavy drinking**

Malt Beer Hard Lemonade ☛ Serving size= fl oz, 335 g; GI= 100 (High); GL= 33.7 (High); Net carb= 33.7 g

Pina Colada Canned ☛ Serving size= 8 fl oz, 266 g; GI= 35 (Low); GL= 25.6 (High); Net carb= 73.2 g

Chocolate-Flavored Soda ☛ Serving size= 8 fl oz, 266 g; GI= 68 (Medium); GL= 19.4 (High); Net carb= 28.5 g

Chocolate Syrup, Made With Whole Milk ☛ Serving size= 1 cup (8 fl oz), 282 g; GI= 57 (Medium); GL= 20.1 (High); Net carb= 35.2 g

Chocolate-Flavor Beverage, Made With Whole Milk ☛ Serving size= 1 serving, 266 g; GI= 77 (High); GL= 23.5 (High); Net carb= 30.5 g

Chocolate-Flavor Beverage, Made With Whole Milk ☛ Serving size= 1 cup (8 fl oz), 266 g; GI= 77 (High); GL= 23.7 (High); Net carb= 30.7 g

Citrus Fruit Juice Drink, Made From Concentrate ☛ Serving size= 8 fl oz, 266 g; GI= 69 (Medium); GL= 73.4 (High); Net carb= 106.4 g

Cocktail Mix Non-Alcoholic Concentrated ☛ Serving size= 4 fl oz, 144 g; GI= 79 (High); GL= 81.5 (High); Net carb= 103.1 g

Cranberry Cocktail ☛ Serving size= 8 fl oz, 266 g; GI= 59 (Medium); GL= 21.2 (High); Net carb= 36 g

Energy Drink ☛ Serving size= 8 fl oz, 266 g; GI= 68 (Medium); GL= 27.1 (High); Net carb= 39.9 g

Energy Drink Full Throttle ☛ Serving size= 8 fl oz, 266 g; GI= 68 (Medium); GL= 21.9 (High); Net carb= 32.1 g

Energy Drink, Amp ☛ Serving size= 8 fl oz, 266 g; GI= 68 (Medium); GL= 21.9 (High); Net carb= 32.1 g

Energy Drink, Monster ☛ Serving size= 8 fl oz, 266 g; GI= 68 (Medium); GL= 20.4 (High); Net carb= 30 g

Energy Drink, Rockstar ☛ Serving size= 8 oz, 266 g; GI= 68 (Medium); GL= 23 (High); Net carb= 33.8 g

Energy Drink, Vault Citrus Flavor ☛ Serving size= 8 fl oz, 266 g; GI= 68 (Medium); GL= 23.5 (High); Net carb= 34.6 g

Fruit Flavored Drink, With Less Than 3% Juice ☛ Serving size= 1 cup (8 fl oz), 238 g; GI= 68 (Medium); GL= 25.9 (High); Net carb= 38.2 g

Fruit Juice Drink, Made With Greater Than 3% Fruit Juice ☛ Serving size= 8 fl oz, 237 g; GI= 68 (Medium); GL= 21 (High); Net carb= 31 g

Fruit Smoothie (average value) ☛ Serving size= 8 fl oz, 266 g; GI= 77 (High); GL= 21.4 (High); Net carb= 27.8 g

Fruit Smoothie, Made With Whole Fruit And Dairy ☛ Serving size= 8 fl oz, 266 g; GI= 77 (High); GL= 21.4 (High); Net carb= 27.8 g

Fruit Smoothie, Made With Whole Fruit No Dairy ☛ Serving size= 8 fl oz, 266 g; GI= 77 (High); GL= 23.3 (High); Net carb= 30.3 g

Fruit Smoothie, Made With Whole Fruit No Dairy And Added

Protein ☛ Serving size= 8 fl oz, 266 g; GI= 77 (High); GL= 22.1 (High); Net carb= 28.8 g

Grape Soda ☛ Serving size= 8 fl oz, 266 g; GI= 68 (Medium); GL= 20.3 (High); Net carb= 29.8 g

Horchata Beverage, Made With Milk ☛ Serving size= 1 cup, 248 g; GI= 45 (Low); GL= 21.5 (High); Net carb= 47.9 g

Horchata Beverage, Made With Water ☛ Serving size= 1 cup, 248 g; GI= 45 (Low); GL= 22.3 (High); Net carb= 49.6 g

Kiwi Strawberry Juice Drink ☛ Serving size= 8 fl oz, 266 g; GI= 68 (Medium); GL= 22.2 (High); Net carb= 32.6 g

Lemonada Limeade (Minute Maid) ☛ Serving size= 8 fl oz, 266 g; GI= 68 (Medium); GL= 24.9 (High); Net carb= 36.6 g

Lemonade (Minute Maid) ☛ Serving size= 8 fl oz, 266 g; GI= 68 (Medium); GL= 21.9 (High); Net carb= 32.1 g

Lemonade, Pink ☛ Serving size= 8 fl oz, 266 g; GI= 89 (High); GL= 115 (High); Net carb= 129.2 g

Lemonade, Pink Made With Water ☛ Serving size= 8 fl oz, 266 g; GI= 68 (Medium); GL= 19.4 (High); Net carb= 28.5 g

Lemonade, White, From Frozen Concentrate ☛ Serving size= 8 fl oz, 266 g; GI= 89 (High); GL= 117.4 (High); Net carb= 131.9 g

Limeade Made With Water, From Frozen Concentrate ☛ Serving size= 8 fl oz, 266 g; GI= 68 (Medium); GL= 24.9 (High); Net carb= 36.7 g

Oatmeal Beverage ☛ Serving size= 1 cup, 248 g; GI= 59 (Medium); GL= 22.5 (High); Net carb= 38.2 g

Orange Breakfast Drink, Ready-To-Drink ☛ Serving size= 8 fl oz, 266 g; GI= 68 (Medium); GL= 23.7 (High); Net carb= 34.8 g

Orange Drink (Breakfast Type) From Frozen Concentrate ☛ Serving size= 8 fl oz, 266 g; GI= 68 (Medium); GL= 70.4 (High); Net carb= 103.5 g

Orange Drink (Breakfast Type), From Frozen Concentrate, Made With Water ☛ Serving size= 8 fl oz, 266 g; GI= 68 (Medium); GL= 20.5 (High); Net carb= 30.1 g

Orange Drink, Canned With Added Vitamin C ☛ Serving size= 8 fl oz, 266 g; GI= 68 (Medium); GL= 22.3 (High); Net carb= 32.8 g

Orange Juice Drink ☛ Serving size= 8 fl oz, 266 g; GI= 68 (Medium); GL= 23.9 (High); Net carb= 35.1 g

Orange Soda ☛ Serving size= 8 fl oz, 266 g; GI= 68 (Medium); GL= 22.2 (High); Net carb= 32.7 g

Orange-Flavor Drink (Breakfast Type), Powder, Made With Water ☛ Serving size= 8 fl oz, 266 g; GI= 68 (Medium); GL= 22.7 (High); Net carb= 33.4 g

Orange-Flavor Drink (Breakfast Type), With Pulp Frozen Concentrate, Made With Water ☛ Serving size= 8 fl oz, 266 g; GI= 68 (Medium); GL= 22.1 (High); Net carb= 32.5 g

Strawberry-Flavor Beverage, Made With Whole Milk, Mix Powder ☛ Serving size= 8 fl oz, 266 g; GI= 68 (Medium); GL= 22.2 (High); Net carb= 32.7 g

DAIRY AND SOY ALTERNATIVES

❄

Cream, heavy, whipped ☛ Serving size: 1 oz (28.35 g); GI= 55.4 (Low); GL= 4.7 (Medium); Net carb= 8.5 g

Cream, whipped, (pressurized container) ☛ Serving size: 1 oz (28.35 g); GI= 55.4 (Medium); GL= 4.7 (Medium); Net carb= 8.5 g

Milk dessert, chocolate ☛ Serving size: 1 cup (136 g); GI= 61 (Medium); GL= 13.3 (Medium); Net carb= 21.8 g

Milk dessert, flavors other than chocolate ☛ Serving size: 1 cup (136 g); GI= 61 (Medium); GL= 13.3 (Medium); Net carb= 21.8 g

Milk dessert, flavors other than chocolate, reduced calorie ☛ Serving size: 1 cup (136 g); GI= 50 (Low); GL= 11.6 (Medium); Net carb= 23.2 g

Milk dessert, flavors other than chocolate ☛ Serving size: 1 cup (136 g); GI= 50 (Low); GL= 11.6 (Medium); Net carb= 23.2 g

Milk shake (average value) ☛ Serving size: 1 cup (226g grams); GI= 44 (Low); GL= 17.9 (Medium); Net carb= 40.7 g

Milk-based fruit drink ☞ Serving size: 1 cup (226g grams); GI= 42.5 (Low); GL= 19.2 (Medium); Net carb= 45.2 g

Milk, oat ☞ Serving size: 1 cup (245 g); GI= 105 (High); GL= 16.8 (Medium); Net carb= 16 g

Milk, rice ☞ Serving size: 1 cup (245 g); GI= 86 (High); GL= 19 (Medium); Net carb= 22.1 g

Mousse chocolate ☞ Serving size: 1 cup (120 g); GI= 69 (Medium); GL= 19.3 (Medium); Net carb= 28 g

Pudding, canned, With chocolate and/or non-chocolate flavors ☞ Serving size: 4 oz (120 g); GI= 44 (Low); GL= 10.6 (Medium); Net carb= 24.1 g

Pudding, canned, tapioca ☞ Serving size: 4 oz (120 g); GI= 64 (Medium); GL= 16.3 (Medium); Net carb= 25.5 g

Pudding, coconut ☞ Serving size: 4 oz (120 g); GI= 44 (Low); GL= 12.7 (Medium); Net carb= 28.9 g

Pudding, rice ☞ Serving size: 4 oz (120 g); GI= 54 (Low); GL= 15.1 (Medium); Net carb= 28 g

Pudding, rice flour, with nuts ☞ Serving size: 4 oz (120 g); GI= 54 (Low); GL= 15.1 (Medium); Net carb= 28 g

Pudding, tapioca, made with milk, from dry mix ☞ Serving size: 4 oz (120 g); GI= 63 (Medium); GL= 16.3 (Medium); Net carb= 26.1 g

Pudding, tapioca, made with milk, from home recipe ☞ Serving size: 4 oz (120 g); GI= 62.5 (Medium); GL= 16.3 (Medium); Net carb= 26.1 g

Pudding, with fruit and vanilla wafers ☞ Serving size: 4 oz (120 g); GI= 86 (High); GL= 15.4 (Medium); Net carb= 26.1 g

LEGUMS AND BEANS

- **Eating raw or undercooked dried beans can lead to food poisoning**

Black Beans, Raw ☛ Serving size= ½ cup, 150 g; GI= 41 (Low); GL= 29.4 (High); Net carb= 71.6 g

Broad beans (Fava), Raw ☛ Serving size= ½ cup, 150 g; GI= 40 (Low); GL= 20 (High); Net carb= 49.9 g

Chickpeas (Garbanzo), Raw ☛ Serving size= ½ cup, 150 g; GI= 36 (Low); GL= 27.4 (High); Net carb= 76.1 g

Cowpeas, Raw ☛ Serving size= ½ cup, 150 g; GI= 50 (Low); GL= 37.1 (High); Net carb= 74.1 g

Green Peas, Raw ☛ Serving size= ½ cup, 150 g; GI= 51 (Low); GL= 30.2 (High); Net carb= 59.1 g

Hyacinth Beans, Raw ☛ Serving size= ½ cup, 150 g; GI= 49 (Low); GL= 25.8 (High); Net carb= 52.7 g

Kidney Beans, All Types, Raw ☛ Serving size= ½ cup, 150 g; GI= 37 (Low); GL= 19.5 (High); Net carb= 52.7 g

Kidney Beans, Raw ☛ Serving size= ½ cup, 150 g; GI= 37 (Low); GL= 25.6 (High); Net carb= 69.1 g

Lima Beans, Raw ☛ Serving size= ½ cup, 150 g; GI= 46 (Low); GL= 30.6 (High); Net carb= 66.6 g

Moth beans, Raw ☛ Serving size= ½ cup, 150 g; GI= 51 (Low); GL= 47.1 (High); Net carb= 92.3 g

Mung Beans, Raw ☛ Serving size= ½ cup, 150 g; GI= 42 (Low); GL= 29.2 (High); Net carb= 69.5 g

Navy Beans, Raw ☛ Serving size= ½ cup, 150 g; GI= 39 (Low); GL= 26.6 (High); Net carb= 68.2 g

Pigeon Peas, Raw ☛ Serving size= ½ cup, 150 g; GI= 31 (Low); GL= 22.2 (High); Net carb= 71.7 g

Pink Beans, Raw ☛ Serving size= ½ cup, 150 g; GI= 37 (Low); GL= 28.6 (High); Net carb= 77.2 g

Pinto Beans, Raw ☛ Serving size= ½ cup, 150 g; GI= 39 (Low); GL= 27.5 (High); Net carb= 70.6 g

Small White Beans, Raw ☛ Serving size= ½ cup, 150 g; GI= 36 (Low); GL= 20.2 (High); Net carb= 56 g

Tofu Yogurt ☛ Serving size= 1 cup, 262 g; GI= 50 (Low); GL= 20.6 (High); Net carb= 41.3 g

White Beans, Raw ☛ Serving size= ½ cup, 150 g; GI= 36 (Low); GL= 24.3 (High); Net carb= 67.6 g

Yardlong Beans,s Raw ☛ Serving size= 1 cup, 167 g; GI= 43 (Low); GL= 36.6 (High); Net carb= 85 g

Yellow Beans, Raw ☛ Serving size= ½ cup, 150 g; GI= 36 (Low); GL= 19.2 (High); Net carb= 53.4 g

FISH & FISH PRODUCTS

Clams—floured, breaded or battered AND baked or fried, baked ☛ Serving size= 3 0z (85 g); GI= 95 (High); GL= 11.9 (Medium)

Crab—soft shell, floured, fried ☛ Serving size= 3 0z (85 g); GI= 95 (High); GL= 11.2 (Medium)

Fish stick—patty, or fillet ☛ Serving size= 3 0z (85 g); GI= 95 (High); GL= 37 (High)

Fish stick—patty, or fillet, floured, breaded or battered AND baked or fried, baked ☛ Serving size= 3 0z (85 g); GI= 95 (High); GL= 37 (High)

Oysters—battered, fried ☛ Serving size= about 12 medium; GI= 95 (High); GL= 11 (Medium)

Oysters—floured or breaded, fried ☛ Serving size= about 12 medium; GI= 95 (High); GL= 11 (Medium)

Scallops—floured, breaded or battered AND baked or fried, baked ☛ Serving size= 3 0z (85 g); GI= 95 (High); GL= 13.7 (Medium)

FRUITS AND FRUITS PRODUCTS

Apple Candied ➙ Serving size= 1 small apple, 198 (g); GI= 44 (Low); GL= 23.3 (High); Net carbs= 53 g

Apples, Canned in Syrup, Drained ➙ Serving size= 1 cup slices, 204 (g); GI= 89 (High); GL= 26.9 (High); Net carbs= 30.3 g

Applesauce, Canned in Syrup, Drained ➙ Serving size= 1 cup, 255 (g); GI= 89 (High); GL= 42.5 (High); Net carbs= 47.7 g

Apricot Dried Cooked Without Sugar ➙ Serving size= 1 cup, 270 (g); GI= 41 (Low); GL= 31.2 (High); Net carbs= 76.1 g

Banana, Baked ➙ Serving size= 1 banana (7-1/4 inch long), 128 (g); GI= 53 (Low); GL= 20.1 (High); Net carbs= 38 g

Banana, Batter-Dipped Fried ➙ Serving size= 1 small, 108 (g); GI= 53 (Low); GL= 21.3 (High); Net carbs= 40.1 g

Banana, unripe ➙ Serving size= 1 cup, mashed, 225 (g); GI= 45 (Low); GL= 20.5 (High); Net carbs= 45.5 g

Breadfruit ➙ Serving size= 1 cup, 220 (g); GI= 65 (Medium); GL= 31.8 (High); Net carbs= 48.9 g

Cherries Sour Red, Canned ☞ Serving size= 1 cup, 261 (g); GI= 73 (High); GL= 54.2 (High); Net carbs= 74.2 g

Cherries Sweet, Canned ☞ Serving size= 1 cup, pitted, 261 (g); GI= 73 (High); GL= 47.1 (High); Net carbs= 64.5 g

Cherries Sweet Juice, Canned ☞ Serving size= 1 cup, pitted, 250 (g); GI= 73 (High); GL= 22.5 (High); Net carbs= 30.8 g

Cranberry Sauce, Canned in Syrup, Drained ☞ Serving size= 1 cup, 277 (g); GI= 77 (High); GL= 83.8 (High); Net carbs= 108.9 g

Cranberry-Orange Relish, Canned in Syrup, Drained ☞ Serving size= 1 cup, 275 (g); GI= 77 (High); GL= 97.8 (High); Net carbs= 127.1 g

Dried Apples ☞ Serving size= 1 cup, 86 (g); GI= 45 (Low); GL= 22.1 (High); Net carbs= 49.2 g

Dried Apricots ☞ Serving size= 1 cup, halves, 130 (g); GI= 41 (Low); GL= 29.5 (High); Net carbs= 71.9 g

Dried Bananas ☞ Serving size= 1 cup, 100 (g); GI= 63 (Medium); GL= 49.4 (High); Net carbs= 78.4 g

Dried Blueberries (Sweetened) ☞ Serving size= 1/4 cup, 40 (g); GI= 73 (High); GL= 21.2 (High); Net carbs= 29 g

Dried Cranberries (Sweetened) ☞ Serving size= 1/4 cup, 40 (g); GI= 73 (High); GL= 22.6 (High); Net carbs= 31 g

Dried Figs ☞ Serving size= 1 cup, 149 (g); GI= 61 (Medium); GL= 49.1 (High); Net carbs= 80.6 g

Dried Peaches ☞ Serving size= 1 cup, halves, 160 (g); GI= 52 (Low); GL= 44.2 (High); Net carbs= 85 g

Dried Pears ☞ Serving size= 1 cup, halves, 180 (g); GI= 54 (Low); GL= 60.5 (High); Net carbs= 112 g

Durian ☞ Serving size= 1 cup, chopped or diced, 243 (g); GI= 49 (Low); GL= 27.7 (High); Net carbs= 56.6 g

Fig Dried Cooked With Sugar ☛ Serving size= 1 cup, 270 (g); GI= 83 (High); GL= 70.7 (High); Net carbs= 85.1 g

Figs, Canned in Syrup, Drained ☛ Serving size= 1 cup, 261 (g); GI= 82 (High); GL= 59.6 (High); Net carbs= 72.7 g

Figs Dried Stewed ☛ Serving size= 1 cup, 259 (g); GI= 61 (Medium); GL= 36.9 (High); Net carbs= 60.5 g

Fruit Cocktail (Grape + Cherry + Peach + Pineapple + Pear), Canned in Syrup ☛ Serving size= 1/2 cup, 130 (g); GI= 79 (High); GL= 22.4 (High); Net carbs= 28.3 g

Fruit Cocktai (Grape + Cherry + Peach + Pineapple + Pear), Canned in Syrup ☛ Serving size= 1 cup, 248 (g); GI= 79 (High); GL= 35.1 (High); Net carbs= 44.4 g

Fruit Cocktail (Grape + Cherry + Peach + Pineapple + Pear), Canned in Syrup ☛ Serving size= 1 cup, 237 (g); GI= 79 (High); GL= 20.3 (High); Net carbs= 25.7 g

Fruit Cocktail (Grape + Cherry + Peach + Pineapple + Pear), Canned in Syrup ☛ Serving size= 1 cup, 242 (g); GI= 79 (High); GL= 26.6 (High); Net carbs= 33.7 g

Fruit Cocktail, Canned Heavy Syrup ☛ Serving size= 1 cup, 214 (g); GI= 79 (High); GL= 28.9 (High); Net carbs= 36.6 g

Fruit Juice, Smoothie, Mighty Mango (Naked Juice) ☛ Serving size= 8 fl oz, 240 (g); GI= 77 (High); GL= 27.7 (High); Net carbs= 36 g

Fruit Juice, Smoothie, Strawberry Banana (Naked Juice) ☛ Serving size= 1 cup, 228 (g); GI= 76 (High); GL= 19.2 (High); Net carbs= 25.2 g

Fruit Salad (Apricot + Cherry + Peach + Pear + Pineapple), Canned in Syrup ☛ Serving size= 1 cup, 259 (g); GI= 68 (Medium); GL= 38.3 (High); Net carbs= 56.4 g

Fruit Salad (Banana + Guava + Pineapple + Papaya) Tropical, Canned in Syrup 🖝 Serving size= 1 cup, 257 (g); GI= 68 (Medium); GL= 36.8 (High); Net carbs= 54.1 g

Golden Seedless Raisins 🖝 Serving size= 1 cup, packed, 165 (g); GI= 53 (Low); GL= 67.1 (High); Net carbs= 126.6 g

Gooseberries, Canned in Syrup, Drained 🖝 Serving size= 1 cup, 252 (g); GI= 78 (High); GL= 32.1 (High); Net carbs= 41.2 g

Grape Juice 🖝 Serving size= 1 cup, 253 (g); GI= 66 (Medium); GL= 24.3 (High); Net carbs= 36.9 g

Grape Juice 🖝 Serving size= 1 cup, 253 (g); GI= 66 (Medium); GL= 24.3 (High); Net carbs= 36.9 g

Grapefruit White Juice, White, Canned, sweetened 🖝 Serving size= 1 cup, 250 (g); GI= 77 (High); GL= 21.2 (High); Net carbs= 27.6 g

Grapefruit Sections, Canned in Syrup, Drained 🖝 Serving size= 1 cup, 254 (g); GI= 77 (High); GL= 29.4 (High); Net carbs= 38.2 g

Guanabana Nectar, Canned 🖝 Serving size= 1 cup, 251 (g); GI= 63 (Medium); GL= 23.5 (High); Net carbs= 37.2 g

Guava Nectar, Canned 🖝 Serving size= 1 cup, 251 (g); GI= 61 (Medium); GL= 23.3 (High); Net carbs= 38.3 g

Jackfruit, Canned Syrup Pack 🖝 Serving size= 1 cup, drained, 178 (g); GI= 81 (High); GL= 33.2 (High); Net carbs= 41 g

Juice, Apple And Grape, Blend 🖝 Serving size= 8 fl oz, 250 (g); GI= 63 (Medium); GL= 19.3 (High); Net carbs= 30.7 g

Juice, Apple Grape And Pear, Blend 🖝 Serving size= 8 fl oz, 250 (g); GI= 63 (Medium); GL= 20.1 (High); Net carbs= 31.9 g

Mango Nectar, Canned in Syrup, Drained 🖝 Serving size= 1 cup, 251 (g); GI= 69 (Medium); GL= 22.2 (High); Net carbs= 32.2 g

Mangosteen, Canned In Syrup 🖝 Serving size= 1 cup, drained, 196 (g); GI= 67 (Medium); GL= 21.2 (High); Net carbs= 31.6 g

THE GLYCEMIC LOAD COUNTER

Orange Pineapple Juice, Blend ☞ Serving size= 8 fl oz, 246 (g); GI= 66 (Medium); GL= 19.5 (High); Net carbs= 29.5 g

Papaya Cooked Or Canned In Sugar Or Syrup ☞ Serving size= 1 cup, 244 (g); GI= 72 (High); GL= 33.6 (High); Net carbs= 46.7 g

Papaya Nectar, Canned ☞ Serving size= 1 cup, 250 (g); GI= 72 (High); GL= 25 (High); Net carbs= 34.8 g

Peach Dried Cooked With Sugar ☞ Serving size= 1 cup, 270 (g); GI= 83 (High); GL= 58 (High); Net carbs= 69.9 g

Peach Nectar, Canned ☞ Serving size= 1 cup, 249 (g); GI= 81 (High); GL= 23.9 (High); Net carbs= 29.5 g

Peaches, Canned in Syrup, Drained ☞ Serving size= 1 cup, halves or slices, 262 (g); GI= 81 (High); GL= 53.2 (High); Net carbs= 65.7 g

Peaches Dried (Sulfured and Stewed), With Added Sugar ☞ Serving size= 1 cup, 270 (g); GI= 83 (High); GL= 54.2 (High); Net carbs= 65.3 g

Peaches Dried (Sulfured and Stewed) Without Added Sugar ☞ Serving size= 1 cup, 258 (g); GI= 52 (Low); GL= 22.8 (High); Net carbs= 43.8 g

Pear Dried Cooked Without Sugar ☞ Serving size= 1 cup, 280 (g); GI= 52 (Low); GL= 51.3 (High); Net carbs= 98.6 g

Pear Nectar, Canned ☞ Serving size= 1 cup, 250 (g); GI= 83 (High); GL= 31.5 (High); Net carbs= 37.9 g

Pears, Canned in Syrup, Drained ☞ Serving size= 1 cup, halves, 247 (g); GI= 83 (High); GL= 21.7 (High); Net carbs= 26.2 g

Pears Dried (Sulfured and Stewed) Without Added Sugar ☞ Serving size= 1 cup, halves, 255 (g); GI= 52 (Low); GL= 36.3 (High); Net carbs= 69.9 g

Pineapple, Canned in Syrup, Drained ☞ Serving size= 1 cup, crushed, sliced, or chunks, 260 (g); GI= 79 (High); GL= 42.5 (High); Net carbs= 53.8 g

Pineapple Juice, Canned Or Bottled, unsweetened ☛ Serving size= 1 cup, 250 (g); GI= 79 (High); GL= 25 (High); Net carbs= 31.7 g

Pineapple Juice unsweetened ☛ Serving size= 1 cup, 250 (g); GI= 79 (High); GL= 24.6 (High); Net carbs= 31.2 g

Plantains Cooked ☛ Serving size= 1 cup, mashed, 200 (g); GI= 40 (Low); GL= 31.3 (High); Net carbs= 78.3 g

Plantains Green Fried ☛ Serving size= 1 cup, 118 (g); GI= 40 (Low); GL= 21.6 (High); Net carbs= 53.9 g

Plums, Canned in Syrup, Drained ☛ Serving size= 1 cup, with pits, yields, 183 (g); GI= 78 (High); GL= 30.9 (High); Net carbs= 39.6 g

Plums Dried Stewed With Added Sugar ☛ Serving size= 1 cup, pitted, 248 (g); GI= 79 (High); GL= 57 (High); Net carbs= 72.1 g

Plums Dried Stewed Without Added Sugar ☛ Serving size= 1 cup, pitted, 248 (g); GI= 50 (Low); GL= 31 (High); Net carbs= 62 g

Pomegranate Juice, Bottled ☛ Serving size= 1 cup, 249 (g); GI= 67 (Medium); GL= 21.7 (High); Net carbs= 32.4 g

Prunes ☛ Serving size= 1 cup, 132 (g); GI= 29 (Low); GL= 34.1 (High); Net carbs= 117.6 g

Prunes, Canned in Syrup, Drained ☛ Serving size= 1 cup, 234 (g); GI= 78 (High); GL= 43.8 (High); Net carbs= 56.2 g

Raisins ☛ Serving size= 1 cup, packed, 165 (g); GI= 59 (Medium); GL= 72.8 (High); Net carbs= 123.5 g

Raisins Cooked ☛ Serving size= 1 cup, 295 (g); GI= 61 (Medium); GL= 100.2 (High); Net carbs= 164.3 g

Rambutan, Canned in Syrup, Drained ☛ Serving size= 1 cup, drained, 150 (g); GI= 77 (High); GL= 23.1 (High); Net carbs= 30 g

Raspberries, Canned in Syrup, Drained ☛ Serving size= 1 cup, 256 (g); GI= 77 (High); GL= 39.5 (High); Net carbs= 51.4 g

Rhubarb, Canned in Syrup, Drained ☛ Serving size= 1 cup, 240 (g); GI= 77 (High); GL= 25.3 (High); Net carbs= 32.8 g

Shredded Coconut Meat (Sweetened) ☛ Serving size= 1 cup, 256 (g); GI= 77 (High); GL= 32.4 (High); Net carbs= 42.1 g

Starfruit Cooked With Sugar ☛ Serving size= 1 cup, 205 (g); GI= 77 (High); GL= 22.4 (High); Net carbs= 29.2 g

Strawberries, Canned in Syrup, Drained ☛ Serving size= 1 cup, 254 (g); GI= 75 (High); GL= 41.6 (High); Net carbs= 55.4 g

Tangerines, Canned in Syrup, Drained ☛ Serving size= 1 cup, 252 (g); GI= 59 (Medium); GL= 23 (High); Net carbs= 39 g

GRAINS AND PASTA

❄

Brown Rice ☛ Serving size= 1 cup (202 g); GI= 68 (Medium); GL= 32.9 (High); Net carb= 48.4 g

Buckwheat Groats Roasted Dry ☛ Serving size= 1 cup (164 g); GI= 55 (Medium); GL= 58.3 (High); Net carb= 106 g

Amaranth Cooked ☛ Serving size= 1 cup (246 g); GI= 95 (High); GL= 38.8 (High); Net carb= 40.8 g

Corn Grain White ☛ Serving size= 1 cup (166 g); GI= 55 (Medium); GL= 67.8 (High); Net carb= 123.3 g

Corn Grain Yellow ☛ Serving size= 1 cup (166 g); GI= 59 (Medium); GL= 65.6 (High); Net carb= 111.2 g

Cornmeal—Degermed Unenriched White or Yellow ☛ Serving size= 1 cup (157 g); GI= 68 (Medium); GL= 80.7 (High); Net carb= 118.6 g

Cornstarch ☛ Serving size= 1 cup (128 g); GI= 97 (High); GL= 112.2 (High); Net carb= 115.7 g

Couscous Cooked ☛ Serving size= 1 cup (157 g); GI= 65 (Medium); GL= 22.3 (High); Net carb= 34.3 g

Couscous Dry ☛ Serving size= 1 cup (173 g); GI= 65 (Medium); GL= 81.4 (High); Net carb= 125.3 g

Couscous Plain Cooked ☛ Serving size= 1 cup (160 g); GI= 65 (Medium); GL= 22.6 (High); Net carb= 34.7 g

Finger millet ☛ Serving size= 1 cup (174 g); GI= 104 (High); GL= 129.1 (High); Net carb= 124.1 g

Foxtail millet ☛ Serving size= 1 cup (174 g); GI= 59 (Medium); GL= 73.2 (High); Net carb= 124.1 g

Japanese Somen Noodles, Dry ☛ Serving size= 1 cup (176 g); GI= 41 (Low); GL= 50.4 (High); Net carb= 122.8 g

Kodo millet ☛ Serving size= 1 cup (174 g); GI= 65 (Medium); GL= 80.7 (High); Net carb= 124.1 g

Little millet ☛ Serving size= 1 cup (174 g); GI= 52 (Low); GL= 64.5 (High); Net carb= 124.1 g

Macaroni Vegetable, fortified Dry ☛ Serving size= 1 cup spiral shaped (84 g); GI= 50 (Low); GL= 29.6 (High); Net carb= 59.3 g

Millet Raw ☛ Serving size= 1 cup (200 g); GI= 53 (Low); GL= 68.2 (High); Net carb= 128.7 g

Noodles Cooked, made with Egg ☛ Serving size= 1 cup (160 g); GI= 55 (Medium); GL= 21.1 (High); Net carb= 38.3 g

Noodles Cooked, made with Rice, Dry ☛ Serving size= 2 oz (57 g); GI= 56 (Medium); GL= 25.1 (High); Net carb= 44.8 g

Noodles Cooked, Whole Grain ☛ Serving size= 1 cup (160 g); GI= 53 (Low); GL= 22.1 (High); Net carb= 41.6 g

Noodles, Cooked ☛ Serving size= 1 cup (160 g); GI= 55 (Medium); GL= 21 (High); Net carb= 38.1 g

Oat Bran ☛ Serving size= 1 cup (94 g); GI= 77 (High); GL= 36.8 (High); Net carb= 47.8 g

Pasta Cooked ☛ Serving size= 1 cup (140 g); GI= 63 (Medium); GL= 25.5 (High); Net carb= 40.4 g

Pasta Cooked, made with Brown Rice Flour, Gluten-Free ☛ Serving size= 1 cup spaghetti not packed (169 g); GI= 71 (High); GL= 36.6 (High); Net carb= 51.5 g

Pasta Cooked, made with Corn And Rice Flour, Gluten-Free ☛ Serving size= 1 cup spaghetti (141 g); GI= 71 (High); GL= 36.7 (High); Net carb= 51.7 g

Pasta Cooked, made with Corn Flour And Quinoa Flour, Gluten-Free ☛ Serving size= 1 cup spaghetti packed (166 g); GI= 70 (High); GL= 32.3 (High); Net carb= 46.2 g

Pasta Cooked, made with Corn, Gluten-Free, Dry ☛ Serving size= 1 cup (105 g); GI= 78 (High); GL= 55.9 (High); Net carb= 71.7 g

Pasta Cooked, Whole Grain ☛ Serving size= 1 cup (140 g); GI= 61 (Medium); GL= 22.2 (High); Net carb= 36.4 g

Pearl millet ☛ Serving size= 1 cup (174 g); GI= 54 (Low); GL= 50.7 (High); Net carb= 94 g

Rice Brown Cooked, Cooked Made With Oil ☛ Serving size= 1 cup (196 g); GI= 56 (Medium); GL= 25.5 (High); Net carb= 45.6 g

Rice Brown Cooked, Made With Butter ☛ Serving size= 1 cup (196 g); GI= 56 (Medium); GL= 25.5 (High); Net carb= 45.6 g

Rice Brown, Long-Grain Raw ☛ Serving size= 1 cup (185 g); GI= 51 (Low); GL= 68.5 (High); Net carb= 134.4 g

Rice Brown, Medium-Grain Raw ☛ Serving size= 1 cup (190 g); GI= 56 (Medium); GL= 77.4 (High); Net carb= 138.3 g

Rice White And Wild, Cooked ☛ Serving size= 1 cup (151 g); GI= 72 (High); GL= 21.9 (High); Net carb= 30.4 g

Rice White Glutinous Cooked ☛ Serving size= 1 cup (174 g); GI= 86 (High); GL= 29.9 (High); Net carb= 34.7 g

Rice White, Cooked Made With Butter ☛ Serving size= 1 cup (163 g); GI= 72 (High); GL= 31.4 (High); Net carb= 43.7 g

Rice White, Cooked Made With Oil ☛ Serving size= 1 cup (163 g); GI= 72 (High); GL= 31.5 (High); Net carb= 43.7 g

Rice White, Long-Grain Parboiled Cooked ☛ Serving size= 1 cup (158 g); GI= 67 (Medium); GL= 26.6 (High); Net carb= 39.7 g

Rice White, Long-Grain Precooked Or Instant, fortified Dry ☛ Serving size= 1 cup (95 g); GI= 56 (Medium); GL= 42.8 (High); Net carb= 76.4 g

Rice White, Long-Grain Regular Cooked ☛ Serving size= 1 cup (158 g); GI= 56 (Medium); GL= 24.6 (High); Net carb= 43.9 g

Rice White, Medium-Grain Cooked Unenriched ☛ Serving size= 1 cup (186 g); GI= 65 (Medium); GL= 34.6 (High); Net carb= 53.2 g

Rice White, Short-Grain Cooked ☛ Serving size= 1 cup (205 g); GI= 72 (High); GL= 42.4 (High); Net carb= 58.9 g

Rye Grain ☛ Serving size= 1 cup (169 g); GI= 59 (Medium); GL= 60.6 (High); Net carb= 102.7 g

Semolina Cooked ☛ Serving size= 1 cup (167 g); GI= 66 (Medium); GL= 76 (High); Net carb= 115.1 g

Sorghum Grain ☛ Serving size= 1 cup (192 g); GI= 66 (Medium); GL= 82.9 (High); Net carb= 125.5 g

Spaghetti Cooked, made with wheat flour ☛ Serving size= 2 oz (57 g); GI= 60 (Medium); GL= 20.4 (High); Net carb= 34 g

Spaghetti Cooked, made with white wheat ☛ Serving size= 2 oz (57 g); GI= 64 (Medium); GL= 21.8 (High); Net carb= 34 g

Spaghetti Cooked, made with whole wheat flour cooked ☛ Serving size= 2 oz (57 g); GI= 65 (Medium); GL= 22.1 (High); Net carb= 34 g

Spelt Cooked ☛ Serving size= 1 cup (194 g); GI= 55 (Medium); GL= 24.1 (High); Net carb= 43.7 g

Tapioca Pearl Dry ☛ Serving size= 1 cup (152 g); GI= 70 (High); GL= 93.4 (High); Net carb= 133.4 g

Triticale ☛ Serving size= 1 cup (192 g); GI= 79 (High); GL= 109.4 (High); Net carb= 138.5 g

Wheat Germ Crude ☛ Serving size= 1 cup (115 g); GI= 59 (Medium); GL= 26.2 (High); Net carb= 44.4 g

Wheat Hard Red Spring ☛ Serving size= 1 cup (192 g); GI= 93 (High); GL= 99.7 (High); Net carb= 107.2 g

Wheat Hard Red Winter ☛ Serving size= 1 cup (192 g); GI= 93 (High); GL= 105.3 (High); Net carb= 113.2 g

Wheat Hard White ☛ Serving size= 1 cup (192 g); GI= 93 (High); GL= 113.7 (High); Net carb= 122.3 g

VEGETABLES

❄

Cassava, cooked ☛ GI= 46 (Low); Serving size= 1 cup (206 g); GL= 34.1 (High); Net carb= 74.2 g

Corn Fritter ☛ GI= 65 (Medium); Serving size= 1 cup (107 g); GL= 26.9 (High); Net carb= 41.3 g

Corn, From Fresh, Canned or Frozen ☛ GI= 48 (Low); Serving size= 1 cup (256 g); GL= 20.7 (High); Net carb= 43.2 g

Corn Sweet White, Cream Style, From Canned ☛ GI= 52 (Low); Serving size= 1 cup (256 g); GL= 22.5 (High); Net carb= 43.3 g

Corn Sweet White, Canned or Boiled Whole Kernel ☛ GI= 52 (Low); Serving size= 1 cup (256 g); GL= 19.6 (High); Net carb= 37.7 g

Corn Sweet Yellow, Cream Style, From Canned or Boiled ☛ GI= 52 (Low); Serving size= 1 cup (256 g); GL= 22.5 (High); Net carb= 43.3 g

Corn White, Cream Style, From Canned or Boiled ☛ GI= 55 (Medium); Serving size= 1 cup (256 g); GL= 24.5 (High); Net carb= 44.5 g

Corn Yellow, Cream Style, From Canned or Boiled ☛ GI= 62 (Medium); Serving size= 1 cup (256 g); GL= 26.8 (High); Net carb= 43.3 g

Starchy Vegetables (Tannier, White Sweet Potato And Yam No Plantain) ☛ GI= 84 (High); Serving size= 1 cup (190 g); GL= 48.8 (High); Net carb= 58.1 g

Starchy Vegetables (Tannier White Sweet Potato And Yam With Green Or Ripe Plantains) ☛ GI= 84 (High); Serving size= 1 cup (195 g); GL= 49.2 (High); Net carb= 58.6 g

Starchy Vegetables (Puerto Rican Style) ☛ GI= 86 (High); Serving size= 1 cup (195 g); GL= 50.4 (High); Net carb= 58.6 g

Sweet Potato Canned ☛ GI= 66 (Medium); Serving size= 1 cup, pieces (250 g); GL= 30.3 (High); Net carb= 45.9 g

Sweet Potato Casserole Or Mashed ☛ GI= 66 (Medium); Serving size= 1 cup (250 g); GL= 25.7 (High); Net carb= 39 g

Sweet Potato Baked ☛ GI= 79 (Medium); Serving size= 1 cup, mashed (328 g); GL= 41.3 (High); Net carb= 52.2 g

White potato ☛ GI= 66 (Medium); Serving size= 1 medium (260 g); GL= 92.5 (High); Net carb= 15.8 g

White potato—baked, peel not eaten ☛ GI= 73 (High); Serving size= 1 medium (260 g); GL= 121.7 (High); Net carb= 19 g

White potato—french fries, breaded or battered ☛ GI= 75 (High); Serving size= 1 medium (260 g); GL= 117.1 (High); Net carb= 17.7 g

White potato—french fries, from fresh or frozen, deep fried ☛ GI= 75 (High); Serving size= 1 medium (260 g); GL= 111 (High); Net carb= 16.7 g

White potato, mashed, made with water, from dry mix ☛ GI= 85 (High); Serving size= 1 medium (260 g); GL= 135.3 (High); Net carb= 18 g

White potato mashed, from dry ☛ GI= 85 (High); Serving size= 1 medium (260 g); GL= 135 (High); Net carb= 18 g

White potato mashed, from fresh ☛ GI= 79 (High); Serving size= 1 medium (260 g); GL= 126 (High); Net carb= 18 g

White potato hash brown, from Fresh, Frozen or dry mix ☛ GI= 75 (High); Serving size= 1 medium (260 g); GL= 132.3 (High); Net carb= 20 g

White potato—home fries ☛ GI= 75 (High); Serving size= 1 medium (260 g); GL= 126.3 (High); Net carb= 19.1 g

HEALTH AND NUTRITION WEBSITES

- **American Diabetes Association:** www.diabetes.org
- **American Heart Association:** www.americanheart.org
- **Centers for Disease Control and Prevention:** www.cdc.gov/diabetes/basics/index.html
- **National Institute of Diabetes and Digestive and Kidney Diseases**: www.niddk.nih.gov/
- **National Institutes of Health:** health.nih.gov
- **Nutrition.gov:** www.nutrition.gov

Made in the USA
Columbia, SC
17 November 2022